to my mother, Emma, who would have been very proud of me
——VERONICA ATKINS

• Contents •

Salads.........................47

Main Courses.........................61

Sauces 155

Dressings 173

• Lose Weight, Look Great, • and Enjoy Your Food

by *Robert C. Atkins*, M.D.

Suppose you love food—everybody does—and yet you have weight to lose and weight to keep off. And you love not just any food, but mouth-watering, rich, and satisfying food. You're facing a dilemma—a choice between looking and feeling great or eating well.

You *can* have both. Using this very special cookbook, food lovers will learn to create sumptuous dishes and lose weight while making garden-variety dieters envious. You will enjoy all the things that other diets told you to avoid. What's more, the recipes in this book have such universal appeal that you can use them for a dinner party and no one will guess you are on a diet—unless, of course, you choose to share with them the "secret" that no one else seems to know:

The secret is the Atkins diet.

The Atkins diet is not just another novelty diet; it is not simply one of your many dieting options. It is so different from other approaches to losing weight that you cannot help but feel "this can't be true!"

But I'll wager that most of you who read my book *Dr. Atkins' New Diet Revolution,* and tried the diet, smile when you hear such disbelief. You know from experience that what I say is true. For those of you not as familiar with it, the Atkins diet is specifically geared to correct the metabolic imbalance that causes people to become overweight.

Excess weight, especially a significant degree of it, represents an identifiable metabolic disorder called hyperinsulinism. Blood tests will show if you have it. And if you do, you can correct it—actually bypass it—by sharply cutting down on your carbohydrate intake. The reason: Insulin floods the bloodstream only when carbohydrates are consumed, so eliminate carbohydrates and you completely bypass your insulin problem. As a hyperinsulinism victim, you are metabolically quite normal unless and until you take in carbohydrates.

Getting your carbohydrate intake down to nearly zero induces your body to put out a biochemical symphony of fat-mobilizing chemicals. When they build up in your bloodstream, as they do whenever you go forty-eight hours or more without carbohydrates, you will normalize your blood sugar, have more energy, and be much less hungry. Because your hunger will be so reduced, the food you eat will fill and satisfy you. And yet, simultaneously, you will be losing weight rather rapidly—at a rate that usually occurs only on some kind of starvation diet. Even more curious, you'll be taking off inches from where you most want to give up unwanted fat.

Despite the medical truth of these principles, we live in an age where the low-fat "fad" diet has become so popular that very few people question it. The low-fat diet has even become the standard diet. Restaurants, cookbook authors, and dietitians, among others, have tried to convince us that a low-fat diet is, or can be made to be, satisfying.

But is food as enjoyable and fulfilling as it was in the "good old days"? Not to me, that's for sure. The restaurants I grew up with don't exist as they did; they don't make the same succulent dishes they used to serve. The delis whose corned beef won "Best in the City" awards years ago now offer a fat-trimmed variant that's not worth eating. And yet the magazines and newspapers rave about this fat-free, stripped-down "cuisine" with such unbridled enthusiasm that I wonder if "gourmet" and "masochist" have now become synonymous. No matter what other recipe books claim, fat-free foods just taste different. There is no delicious substitute for heavy cream, pâté, or bacon. The low-fat creations just don't work because fat creates, translates, and intensifies flavor, and is what makes you feel sated and full. Your body can't be fooled, nor can your taste buds.

For any diet to be successful, it must be a lifetime eating plan. The metabolic imbalance leading to being overweight doesn't go away, so your diet must master it forever. But other cookbooks expect you to live the rest of your life eating bland fat-free foods. Imagine a life without real butter, real cream, real steak. That is why so many other diets fail. The requirements are so stringent and so boring that no one can bear to stay on them.

This book is designed to be a guide for you, a guide to a revolution in eating—a new diet revolution. Using the recipes in this extraordinary book, you will cook and enjoy eating real foods. Written by low-carbohydrate gourmet Veronica Atkins, my wife, these recipes rival those of any restaurant or gourmet magazine. When you taste her creations, you will become fully aware of just what you have been missing. You will be clued into a most fascinating paradox: Diet food can be better, richer, and more sumptuous than most everyday foods.

And because sitting down to dinner together is precious time for any family, Veronica has ingeniously created mouth-watering meals that can be prepared in thirty minutes or less. This will allow you to focus on the good food and wonderful companionship when enjoying meals with your family and friends. And isn't that what eating should really be about?

by Veronica Atkins

Dr. Atkins and I developed this book not only to whet your appetite but to give you the know-how to lead the low-carbohydrate life. We never want you to feel as if you're on a diet. We want you to enjoy the varied and luxurious cuisine that a low-carbohydrate diet offers.

This book is also designed for the busy home cook, so all the recipes can be made in thirty minutes or less. These dishes are satisfying as well as delicious, nutritious as well as substantial, and easy as well as flexible. In these recipes I did not skimp on flavors or ingredients because I didn't have to, and my sentiments about food would not allow me to.

Throughout my life, food has played a pivotal role. Growing up in postwar Europe, food was very scarce, but my family still enjoyed wonderfully creative dishes. As an opera singer I lived in many countries with unique culinary traditions and discovered many new foods and flavors. Then in the United States I met a kindred spirit, a revolutionary doctor, who saw food as something much more powerful than mere sustenance.

My marriage and my work with Dr. Atkins and his low-carbohydrate diet were a natural continuation of my lifelong love affair with food. I began to create low-carbohydrate recipes that were easy and delicious. All of our friends would ask me for my secrets. But with the low-carbohydrate diet, you don't need some secret, complicated way of cooking. Just a few simple steps can start you on the diet of a lifetime.

You will be amazed how easy it is to modify your own cooking style to create a low-carbohydrate menu. Main-course dishes are wonderfully easy to tailor to the low-carbohydrate diet because most of them are already protein-based. The recipes included in this book are some of my favorites, and after working with them, you will soon learn how to modify your own favorite main-course recipes to make them perfect for the diet.

Vegetable dishes are almost as easy to modify to the low-carbohydrate diet. Just keep handy a list of the permissible vegetables. I have also tried to make the vegetable dishes extra flavorful and luxurious, and so they can often stand on their own as the centerpiece of a meal.

Breads and desserts are a bit harder to modify but not impossible. By testing different substitute ingredients, I have found the best combinations to create delicious low-carbohydrate recipes.

But this book isn't really about dieting. It is a book about food, real food, sumptuous food. I encourage you to explore your palate, try new flavors, and see cooking as fun, not a chore. Sadly, the art of the kitchen has diminished, and because we are all so pressed for time, prepackaged foods wait on the shelves as a quick-fix answer. But people are demanding a change! They are sick and tired (literally) of the invented foods that contain no fat, no flavor, and no pleasure. Luxurious foods with rich flavors are now what we demand. And there is just no other diet in existence more suited for the rediscovery of home cooking. This book will change your perception of cooking and dieting. You will come to view them not as a brief experiment but as a lifelong practice, not as a painful experience but as a constant pleasure.

QUICK AND EASY KITCHEN STRATEGIES

When you cook every day, your kitchen has to be simple and efficient. And taking control of your pantry and refrigerator makes dieting much easier, too. The following are some practical suggestions to get your kitchen up and running for the rest of your low-carbohydrate life.

Clean House

Get rid of the temptations! You probably have a lot of carbohydrates lurking about your kitchen: crackers, bread crumbs, baked beans, cookies, skim milk, jams, and so forth. This does not necessarily mean that you have to throw them all away—or that you should have a final binge—because others in your home may not be joining you on the diet. The recipes in this book are appropriate for the whole family, but anyone who chooses to can add a few carbohydrates to the side of the main course you've prepared.

But do gather up the carbohydrate foods and put them in a separate part of your pantry and refrigerator. When you are cooking the wonderful recipes in this book, you'll want your shelves to be full of the delicious, low-carbohydrate foods you can use with ease. If all members of your household are going on the diet or you live alone, of course you can get rid of all those high-carbohydrate temptations.

Managing Your Week

With a little planning you can create the simple building blocks for your week's dining. If you prepare a few sauces at the start of the week, you can combine them with protein staples (chicken, beef, fish, and so on, see page 211 for a complete list) or leftovers. And you'll end up with a variety of flavorful meals for the whole week. Of course, if you prefer, all of the sauces can be made at the last moment.

For example, if you make Cilantro-Lime Pesto (page 161), you can serve it with grilled chicken the first day, use it in an omelet with feta the following day, and then add a tablespoon of it to your tuna salad on another day. So if you make as few as three sauces at the beginning of the week, your meals are practically set.

Shopping

At the base of the Atkins diet are fresh, wholesome ingredients, most of which you can purchase in your local supermarket. In fact, shopping for this diet can make your visits to the supermarket shorter and simpler. In our experience the fresh ingredients are found on the perimeter of the supermarket, where meats, vegetables, and dairy are located. The store's middle shelves are usually filled with over-processed high-carbohydrate foods, and now you can just skip past them. When you buy your food, try to buy fresh, natural, unprocessed food, and whenever possible, try to find organic foods that are grown without hormones and pesticides.

Once a month or so you may need to go to a specialty or health-food store for specific ingredients. If you stock up, you'll have what you need for daily use. If you cannot find some of the ingredients locally, most are available by mail order.

Ordering Supplies by Mail

Some of you may not be able to find some of these ingredients in your local store. For up-to-date mail-order information on items such as Atkins Bake Mix, soy flour, tofu flour, whey protein, and Stevia, you can call 1-888-DR ATKINS.

Equipment

A quick and easy kitchen should have some quick and easy equipment. These few additions to your basic store of pots and pans can greatly reduce both preparation and cooking time.

FOOD PROCESSOR: A must for any kitchen, it allows you to create innumerable dishes and frees you from depending on bottled dressing, sauces, and canned soups.

R AMEKINS : Great for baking individual portions, they reduce cooking time.

FLAMEPROOF SKILLET : Offers the convenience of transferring a dish directly from the stovetop to the oven.

MUFFIN TINS : Reduces the cooking time needed for quick and easy breads.

DOUBLE BOILER : Lets you make delicate sauces, or melt cheese.

ENAMEL SKILLET : This is Dr. Atkins' personal favorite cooking tool.

HIDDEN CARBOHYDRATES

Not that long ago it was hard to figure out the real carbohydrate content and count of many foods. But now, with labeling laws in place, the "carbohydrate grams per serving" is clearly shown in the nutritional description of all processed foods. In assessing carbohydrates, make sure you consider your serving size (usually shown on the top of the label). All too often the serving size, for which carbohydrate grams are measured, is only a small portion of the whole. This can be very misleading, so read all labels carefully. As a rule, when a label states that a portion is "less than 1 gram" of carbohydrate, you should count it as a full gram because it could be up to .99 of a gram. When it comes to counting carbohydrates, it's always better to overestimate.

You may be surprised at the foods that have carbohydrates stuffed in them. Here are some you should watch out for:

- Luncheon meats, bottled salad dressings, margarine, imitation mayonnaise, ketchup, relish, pickles, and diet cheeses. These often have sugars or starches added.

- Prepared gravies and sauces. These often have starches as thickeners or sugars as sweeteners.

- Other carbohydrate-laden sweeteners, such as sorbitol, mannitol, other hexitols; as well as other sweeteners with the suffix *-ose,* such as maltose and fructose. Read "sugar-free" labels carefully. Products may not contain sugar, but they may still have these sweeteners. Also be alert to "no sugar added" labels because these products may include natural sugars.

- Dairy products. Remember that, as a rule, the lower the fat content of a milk product, the higher its carbohydrate grams. Use cream, not skim milk; use sour cream, not yogurt.

- Chewing gum, breath mints, cough drops, and cough syrups. These often contain sugar and carbohydrates. Be wary.

- "Low-fat" and "fat-free" foods. Cutting fat usually means that more sugars and carbohydrates have been added.

HINTS FOR MODIFYING OTHER RECIPES TO THE LOW-CARBOHYDRATE DIET

- Refer to the Quick and Easy Low-Carbohydrate Food List in the back of this book (pages 211–213) as a guide to foods you can eat on the Atkins diet.

- For dredging, use Atkins Bake Mix, soy flour, tofu flour, or whey protein instead of flour.

- Use cauliflower, not potatoes, to thicken soups.

- Use cream or egg yolks, not flour, to thicken sauces.

- Onions have carbohydrates, so try to use minimal amounts of them or add a bit of onion powder instead.

- When a recipe contains several vegetables, refer to the list of Low-Carbohydrate Vegetables (page 212). Omit the vegetables from the recipe that are not on the list and substitute ones that are.

- Change the ratio of vegetables to meat. In a given recipe, cut back on the amount of vegetables and increase the amount of meat.

- Use quick and easy Breading I, II, or III (pages 190–192) instead of the traditional kind. For recipes that call for breading to be sprinkled on top of something, you can try using a mixture of chopped nuts and cheese.

- For spreads and dips, use elegant whole endive leaves, hard-boiled eggs, or plain frittatas, cut into wedges, or pork rinds instead of crackers and bread.

- Most baked egg dishes don't need a crust. Just butter your pan well and pour the eggs directly into it.

- Experiment with sugar substitutes. We suggest using a combination of them because when they are mixed together, sweeteners create a synergistic effect. Therefore, less is needed. We recommend not using Equal or aspartame in cooking or baking; they lose their sweetness when heated.*

- Don't assume any food is low carbohydrate. Read all labels and invest in a carbohydrate counter. And always check foods first.

* Although most published scientific studies have proclaimed aspartame (NutraSweet, Equal) to be safe, clinical experience has often indicated otherwise. Headaches, irritability, and failure to lose weight or to control blood glucose have all been reported, as well as cross reactions in those who cannot tolerate monosodium glutamate (MSG). Consult with your local doctor if you have any concern about your use of aspartame. The best advice may be to use it sparingly, preferably blending it with other sweeteners.

QUICK AND EASY GUIDE TO
THE *QUICK AND EASY*
NEW DIET COOKBOOK

This cookbook is a companion to *Dr. Atkins' New Diet Revolution,* which provides an in-depth explanation of the four phases of the Atkins low-carbohydrate diet and the scientific principles behind it. As you use this cookbook, keep in mind that success on the Atkins diet depends on your accurately counting the total carbohydrate grams consumed per day. You should therefore determine how many carbohydrate grams you have in each meal, and to ensure that you do not exceed your carbohydrate limit, consider any additional carbohydrates you consume in snacks or desserts. We have created recipes in this book that are appropriate to each phase of your diet. Following are some brief guidelines to keep in mind when choosing a recipe:

During the *Induction Phase,* you should consume no more than 20 grams of carbohydrate a day. But remember, you are in this phase for only two weeks.

During the *Ongoing Weight Loss Phase,* you need to find your own "Critical Carbohydrate Level," as explained in *Dr. Atkins' New Diet Revolution.* For the average dieter, this level is 30 to 50 grams each day.

During the *Pre-maintenance Phase,* weight loss is slowed considerably.

During the *Maintenance Phase,* the goal is simply to maintain your ideal (goal) weight.

In both the Pre-maintenance Phase and the Maintenance Phase, you can use those recipes with the highest carbohydrate gram counts.

Don't forget to think in terms of total carbohydrate grams per meal and total carbohydrate grams per day.

If you find our recipes as useful as we think you will, you should also enjoy the recipes in *Dr. Atkins' New Diet Revolution* and *Dr. Atkins' New Diet Cookbook.*

Hors d'oeuvres, Appetizers, and Snacks

•

Guacamole

Zucchini Rolls with Chèvre

Artichoke Hearts Wrapped in Bacon

Two-Cheese Spread

Baked Goat Cheese and Ricotta Custards

Deviled Eggs

Curried Stuffed Eggs

Smoked Salmon Rolls

Chicken Liver Pâté with Cloves

· Guacamole ·

Guacamole is not just a dip anymore. This spicy Mexican specialty makes a tasty topping for an omelet or a colorful bed for grilled chicken.

> TOTAL CARBOHYDRATES: 20.5 grams
>
> PER SERVING: 10.3 grams

1 Haas avocado, cut into
   ³/₈-inch cubes
¹/₃ cup finely chopped onion
¹/₃ cup chopped tomato
1 teaspoon chopped jalapeño
   (optional)

3 tablespoons chopped fresh
   cilantro
1 tablespoon fresh lime juice
1 tablespoon olive oil
salt and pepper to taste

• **Combine the avocado, onion, tomato, jalapeño, if using, cilantro, lime juice, oil, salt, and pepper in a bowl, and mix gently. Serve immediately or store, covered, in the refrigerator for up to 2 days.**

Serves 2

• Zucchini Rolls with Chèvre •

Zucchini rolls make a lovely appetizer or hors d'oeuvre. You can substitute other soft cheeses, such as cream cheese or ricotta, for the chèvre.

> TOTAL CARBOHYDRATES: *13 grams*
>
> PER SERVING: *6.5 grams*

2 large zucchini, cut
    lengthwise into six
    ³/₈-inch-thick slices
2 tablespoons olive oil
1¹/₂ ounces chèvre cheese,
    softened

2 tablespoons chopped tomato
2 tablespoons chopped fresh
    flat-leaf parsley
salt and pepper to taste

●   **Preheat the grill or broiler.**
    Brush the zucchini slices with the oil and grill or broil for 2 to 3 minutes on each side, or until lightly browned. Let the zucchini cool slightly and spread each slice with 1¹/₂ teaspoons of chèvre. Top with 1 teaspoon of chopped tomato and 1 teaspoon of parsley, and season with salt and pepper. Roll up the zucchini slices, jelly-roll style, and secure with toothpicks. Serve immediately.

Serves 2

Artichoke Hearts Wrapped in Bacon

These easy-to-prepare artichoke hearts are fabulous hors d'oeuvres or snacks.

> TOTAL CARBOHYDRATES: *18.2 grams*
>
> PER SERVING: *1.5 per piece*

¼ pound thinly sliced bacon
one 14-ounce can artichoke
*   hearts, drained, or*
*   1 package (10½ ounces)*
*   frozen artichoke hearts,*
*   thawed; cut in half*

* **Preheat the broiler.**
  Cut the bacon slices in half, place on a baking sheet, and broil for 3 minutes. Let the bacon cool.
  When the bacon is cool enough to handle, wrap each artichoke half in a piece of bacon, broiled side facing inward, and secure with a toothpick. Broil 4 to 5 minutes, or until the bacon is brown and crisp. Serve immediately.

Serves 2

• Two-Cheese Spread •

This tangy cheese spread is great on our Sesame Sour Cream Muffins (page 186). You can also serve it melted over sautéed vegetables to create a luscious side dish.

TOTAL CARBOHYDRATES:
.76 gram per ¾ cup

⅓ cup grated sharp cheddar cheese

⅓ cup grated Monterey Jack cheese

4 tablespoons (½ stick) butter

1½ teaspoons olive oil

• **Combine the cheddar, Monterey Jack, and butter in a small saucepan (preferably nonstick) and cook, stirring, over low heat about 3 minutes, until the cheese mixture becomes smooth and thick. Pour the oil into a small bowl or ramekin and pour the cheese mixture over it. Cover and chill for 10 minutes. Store in the refrigerator for up to 5 days.**

Makes about ¾ cup

• Baked Goat Cheese and •
Ricotta Custards

Baked in individual ramekins, these savory custards are wrapped in spinach leaves. Serve them on mixed greens as a first course or luncheon entree.

> TOTAL CARBOHYDRATES: *11.4 grams*
>
> PER SERVING: *5.7 grams*

butter for greasing the
    ramekins
½ cup whole-milk ricotta
    cheese
3 ounces fresh goat cheese
1½ tablespoons grated
    Parmesan cheese
1½ tablespoons coarsely
    chopped walnuts

1 tablespoon chopped fresh
    basil leaves
1 egg, lightly beaten
salt and pepper to taste
6 large spinach leaves,
    stemmed and washed

- **Preheat the oven to 350°F.**
Generously butter two 5-ounce ramekins.
Combine the ricotta, goat cheese, Parmesan, walnuts, basil, egg, salt, and pepper in a bowl and mix well. Line each ramekin with 3 spinach leaves. Add the cheese mixture to the ramekins, filling them ¾ full, and bake for 30 minutes. Let the ramekins cool for 5 minutes.

To serve, place a small serving plate on top of each ramekin and turn the ramekins upside down, cutting away any spinach that overlaps the rims. Tap the bottom of the ramekins, then remove them, releasing the custards. The ramekins should slide off easily. Serve immediately.

Serves 2

• Deviled Eggs •

These tangy stuffed eggs make a surefire appetizer or snack. You may want to double or triple the recipe when entertaining—they'll disappear very quickly.

> TOTAL CARBOHYDRATES: *2.4 grams*
>
> PER SERVING: *1.2 grams*

3 hard-boiled eggs
2 teaspoons minced capers
1 tablespoon minced celery
1 tablespoon minced scallion
    (white part only)
1 ounce boiled ham, minced
1 tablespoon mayonnaise

½ teaspoon Dijon mustard
salt and pepper to taste
paprika for garnish (optional)
chopped fresh flat-leaf parsley
    or chopped fresh dill for
    garnish (optional)

• **Cut the eggs in half, remove the yolks, and place them in a bowl. Reserve the whites. Add the capers, celery, scallion, ham, mayonnaise, mustard, salt, and pepper to the egg yolks and mix well.**

Divide the yolk mixture evenly among the reserved whites, mounding it slightly. Garnish the deviled eggs with paprika and parsley if desired. Serve immediately or store, covered, in the refrigerator for up to 1 day.

Serves 2

• Curried Stuffed Eggs •

Keep these delicious stuffed eggs on hand to serve as hors d'oeuvres or snacks. The recipe easily lends itself to doubling or tripling.

> TOTAL CARBOHYDRATES: .9 gram
>
> PER SERVING: .5 gram

4 hard-boiled eggs
1 teaspoon Dijon mustard
1 tablespoon mayonnaise

$^1/_2$ teaspoon curry powder
pinch of cayenne pepper
salt and black pepper to taste

• Cut the eggs in half, remove the yolks, and place them in a bowl. Reserve the whites. Add the mustard, mayonnaise, curry powder, cayenne, salt, and black pepper to the egg yolks and mix well. Divide the yolk mixture evenly among the reserved whites, mounding it slightly. Serve immediately or store, covered, in the refrigerator for up to 1 day.

Serves 2

• Smoked Salmon Rolls •

These elegant hors d'oeuvres are delicate and flavorful. Serve them with a drizzling of lemon juice if desired.

> TOTAL CARBOHYDRATES: 1.7 grams
>
> PER SERVING: .9 gram

2 ounces thinly sliced smoked
    salmon
about 2 tablespoons
    Horseradish Cream
    (page 168)

about 1 tablespoon capers
1 teaspoon chopped fresh dill

• Cut the salmon into 1-inch strips. Put a small dollop of horseradish cream on one end of the salmon strip and top with a caper and a sprinkling of dill. Roll up the salmon strips, jelly-roll style, and secure with toothpicks. Serve immediately.

Serves 2

• Chicken Liver Pâté with Cloves •

Pâté is an elegant hors d'oeuvre as well as an easy, delicious snack. For a sumptuous twist on the traditional deviled egg, try using this chicken liver pâté as a filling for hard-boiled egg whites.

TOTAL CARBOHYDRATES:
4.5 grams per ¾ cup

¼ pound chicken livers
2 tablespoons butter, softened
¼ teaspoon mustard powder
⅛ teaspoon ground cloves
1 tablespoon grated onion

pinch of cayenne pepper
salt and black pepper to taste
2 teaspoons dry sherry
(optional)

• Place the chicken livers in a saucepan. Add enough water to just cover them, bring to a boil, and lower the heat. Simmer the livers, covered, for 15 to 20 minutes, or until tender. Drain the livers and transfer to a food processor.

Add the butter, mustard powder, cloves, onion, cayenne, salt, black pepper, and sherry, if using. Puree, scraping down the side, for 1 minute, or until smooth. Transfer the pâté to a bowl and chill for 10 minutes. Serve immediately or store, covered, in the refrigerator for up to 3 days.

Makes about ¾ cup

Soups

•

Cucumber Dill Soup
Spinach and Clam Soup
Roasted Pepper Soup
French Onion Soup Gratinée
Asparagus and Leek Soup
Cream of Watercress Soup
Avocado Soup
Blue Cheese and Bacon Soup

• Cucumber Dill Soup •

During the warm-weather months we keep a container of this refreshing soup in the refrigerator for a quick afternoon snack.

> TOTAL CARBOHYDRATES:
>
> 11.2 grams per 2 cups

1 tablespoon olive oil
⅓ cup chopped onion
1 large cucumber, peeled,
  seeded, and cut into ½-
  inch slices
1 cup chicken stock

1 tablespoon balsamic vinegar
½ cup chopped fresh dill
salt and pepper to taste
sour cream as an
  accompaniment
  (optional)

● Heat the oil in a large saucepan over medium-high heat until hot but not smoking. Add the onion and sauté, stirring, for 2 minutes. Add the cucumbers and stock, and bring to a boil. Lower the heat, cover, and simmer for 10 minutes. Stir in the vinegar, dill, salt, and pepper.

Transfer the mixture to a food processor and puree for 1 minute, or until smooth. Serve chilled with the sour cream if desired.

Makes about 2 cups

• Spinach and Clam Soup •

All the ingredients for this full-flavored soup are available year-round. It makes an appetizing starter for Broiled Marinated Lamb Chops (page 117).

> TOTAL CARBOHYDRATES:
>
> 32.3 grams per 3 cups

2 strips bacon, cut into
    1-inch pieces
2 oil-packed anchovy fillets,
    chopped
½ small onion, chopped
1 small clove garlic, minced
2 cups chicken stock

half of a 10½-ounce package
    frozen spinach, thawed
    and squeezed dry
¾ cup chopped fresh or
    canned clams
¾ cup heavy cream
salt and pepper to taste

• Place the bacon, anchovy fillets, onion, and garlic in a large saucepan. Cook over medium heat, stirring, for 3 minutes, or until the bacon begins to brown. Add the stock and bring to a boil. Stir in the spinach, clams, and cream, and return to a boil. Add the salt and pepper, lower the heat, and simmer for 4 minutes. Serve immediately.

Makes about 3 cups

• *Roasted Pepper Soup* •

Tangy Parmesan and sweet roasted peppers make this soup flavorful and satisfying.

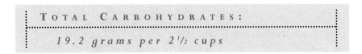

TOTAL CARBOHYDRATES:

19.2 grams per 2½ cups

2 tablespoons olive oil
1 celery stalk, trimmed and
    chopped
⅓ cup chopped onion
1 clove garlic, minced
2 roasted yellow or red
    peppers (see procedure on
    page 150), peeled,
    seeded, and chopped

1½ cups chicken stock
⅓ cup heavy cream
salt and black pepper to taste
¼ cup grated Parmesan cheese

• Heat the oil in a skillet over moderate heat until hot but not smoking. Add the celery, onion, and garlic, and cook, stirring occasionally, about 5 minutes, until the celery is soft. Add the peppers and stock. Bring to a boil, then lower the heat and simmer for 3 minutes.

Transfer the mixture to a food processor. Add the cream, salt, and pepper, and process about 45 seconds, until smooth. Ladle the soup into 2 serving bowls and sprinkle with Parmesan. Serve immediately.

Makes about 2½ cups

• French Onion Soup Gratinée •

This comforting soup is one of our all-time favorites. Serve it with Mixed Green Salad with Warm Bacon Dressing (page 56) for a cozy, satisfying supper.

TOTAL CARBOHYDRATES: 17 grams
PER SERVING: 8.5 grams

1 tablespoon olive oil
1 medium onion, thinly sliced
one 14-ounce can chicken
    stock
1 tablespoon Worcestershire
    sauce

½ cube of beef bouillon
2 tablespoons dry sherry
¼ cup grated Parmesan cheese
salt and pepper to taste
2 ounces Swiss cheese, grated
nutmeg to taste

• **Preheat the broiler.**

Heat the oil in a large saucepan over medium-low heat until hot but not smoking. Add the onion and cook, stirring occasionally, for 10 minutes, or until golden. Raise the heat to medium-high and add the chicken stock, Worcestershire sauce, bouillon, and sherry. Bring to a boil, then lower the heat and simmer for 3 minutes. Add the Parmesan, salt, and pepper, and simmer for another 3 minutes.

Transfer the soup to 2 large flameproof bowls and top each with half of the Swiss cheese. Broil for 3 to 4 minutes, until the cheese is melted and golden brown. Sprinkle the soup with nutmeg and serve immediately.

Serves 2

• Asparagus and Leek Soup •

Here's a simple soup in which the taste of the vegetables really comes through. Recipes often call for a soup such as this to be strained, but I prefer the earthy texture of the more rustic version.

> TOTAL CARBOHYDRATES:
>
> 16.6 grams per 3 1/2 cups

2 tablespoons butter
1 leek (white part only),
    halved lengthwise,
    washed well, and
    chopped

3/4 pound asparagus, cut into
    1/2-inch pieces
2 cups chicken stock
1/3 cup heavy cream
salt and pepper to taste

• Heat the butter in a large saucepan over medium-high heat until the foam subsides. Add the leek and sauté, stirring, for 2 minutes. Add the asparagus and sauté, stirring, for 1 minute. Add the stock to the pan and bring to a boil. Lower the heat, cover, and simmer for 8 to 10 minutes, or until the asparagus is tender.

Transfer the mixture to a food processor. Add the cream, salt, and pepper, and puree for 1 minute, or until smooth. Serve immediately.

Makes about 3 1/2 cups

• Cream of Watercress Soup •

Because the watercress is only slightly cooked, it gives this soup a fresh, peppery flavor. Serve it as a first course with Veal Saltimbocca (page 123).

TOTAL CARBOHYDRATES:

12.6 grams per 2 cups

2 tablespoons butter
⅓ cup chopped onion
1 cup chicken stock
¾ cup chopped cauliflower

2 bunches watercress, stemmed
⅓ cup heavy cream
salt and pepper to taste
nutmeg to taste

• Heat the butter in a large saucepan over medium-high heat until the foam subsides. Add the onion and sauté, for 5 minutes, stirring occasionally. Add the stock and cauliflower, and bring to a boil. Lower the heat, cover, and simmer for 10 minutes. Turn off the heat and add the watercress. Cover and let stand for 5 minutes, stirring once.

Transfer the mixture to a food processor. Add the cream, salt, pepper, and nutmeg, and puree for 1 minute, or until smooth. Serve warm or chilled.

Makes 2 cups

• Avocado Soup •

Simple and delicate, this creamy soup makes a sublime starter for Rack of Lamb with Brussels Sprouts (page 119).

> ### TOTAL CARBOHYDRATES:
> 14.2 grams per 2 cups

1 tablespoon butter
1 scallion (white part only), chopped
1 1/2 cups chicken stock
1 Haas avocado, peeled, pitted, and drizzled with lemon juice

1/3 cup heavy cream
salt and pepper to taste

• Heat the butter in a skillet over medium heat until the foam subsides. Add the scallion and cook, stirring occasionally, for 2 minutes, or until translucent. Add 1 cup of the stock, bring to a boil, then lower the heat and simmer for 3 minutes.

Meanwhile, blend the avocado, cream, and remaining 1/2 cup of stock in a food processor until smooth. Add the avocado mixture to the skillet and cook over medium heat, stirring occasionally, for 2 minutes, or until heated through. Season with salt and pepper, and serve.

Makes about 2 cups

• Blue Cheese and Bacon Soup •

Cheese soups are especially savory, and this one is made even more delicious with the addition of the smoky flavor of bacon. If you are not a fan of blue cheese, you can substitute an equal amount of grated cheddar.

> TOTAL CARBOHYDRATES:
>
> 9.4 grams per 2 cups

2 tablespoons butter
1 leek (white part only), halved lengthwise, washed well, and chopped
1 cup sliced mushrooms
½ cup chopped cauliflower
1½ cups chicken stock
2½ ounces blue cheese, crumbled
6 strips bacon, cooked and crumbled

• Heat the butter in a large saucepan over medium heat until the foam subsides. Add the leek, mushrooms, and cauliflower. Cover and cook, stirring occasionally, for 5 minutes. Add the stock and bring to a boil. Lower the heat, cover, and simmer for 10 minutes.

Transfer the mixture to a food processor. Add the blue cheese and puree for 1 minute, or until smooth. Serve immediately with the crumbled bacon on top.

Makes about 2 cups

Salads

•

Orange Daikon Salad

Fennel Salad with Parmesan

Endive Salad with Walnuts and Roquefort

Walnut Coleslaw

Celery Root Salad

Red Cabbage Salad with Feta and Dill

Greek Salad

Mixed Green Salad with Warm Bacon Dressing

Warm Spinach Salad with Bacon and Pine Nuts

Cucumber and Tomato Salad with Mortadella

Bacon and Cabbage Salad

• Orange Daikon Salad •

Crisp, light daikon radish is a perfect ingredient for an easy, refreshing salad. If you can't find daikon, you can substitute jicama for an equally pleasing texture.

> TOTAL CARBOHYDRATES: 9.4 grams
>
> PER SERVING: 4.7 grams

2 cups peeled and sliced
    daikon radish or jicama
    (available at specialty
    produce markets and
    some supermarkets)

2 tablespoons sunflower oil
1 tablespoon red wine vinegar
1 teaspoon grated orange zest
salt to taste

• **Place the daikon in a bowl. In another bowl, whisk together the oil, vinegar, orange zest, and salt until the dressing is well blended. Pour the dressing over the daikon, toss the salad well, and serve immediately.**

Serves 2

• Fennel Salad with Parmesan •

This is one of my favorite summer salads. The flavors are clean and fresh, and the Parmesan gives it just the right saltiness. For an elegant presentation, use a vegetable peeler to shave the Parmesan into paper-thin slices.

> TOTAL CARBOHYDRATES: *8.6 grams*
>
> PER SERVING: *4.3 grams*

1 tablespoon white wine
   vinegar
3 tablespoons olive oil
salt and pepper to taste
1 tablespoon chopped fresh
   dill
1 tablespoon chopped fresh
   flat-leaf parsley

4 small fennel bulbs, halved
   lengthwise, cored, and
   very thinly sliced
8 shavings of Parmesan cheese
   or 2 tablespoons grated
   Parmesan cheese

• Place the vinegar, oil, salt, pepper, dill, and parsley in a small bowl. Whisk until the dressing is smooth. Place the fennel in a large bowl. Add the dressing and toss gently. Divide the salad between 2 serving plates and serve with the Parmesan.

Serves 2

· Endive Salad with Walnuts ·
and Roquefort

The pretty presentation of this salad makes it ideal for a special-occasion meal. You can double or triple the recipe as needed.

> TOTAL CARBOHYDRATES: 10.7 grams
>
> PER SERVING: 5.4 grams

2 tablespoons olive oil
1 teaspoon fresh lemon juice
1 teaspoon fresh orange juice
1 teaspoon grated orange zest
1/3 cup crumbled Roquefort or
    other blue cheese
salt and pepper to taste

1 plump head of endive, leaves
    separated, washed well,
    and spun dry
1/3 cup chopped walnuts,
    lightly toasted (see Hint
    on page 163)

• Whisk together the oil, lemon juice, orange juice, orange zest, Roquefort, salt, and pepper in a small bowl. (If the cheese clumps, mash it with a fork.) Arrange the endive leaves on a serving plate like the spokes of a wheel. Pour the Roquefort dressing over the endive and sprinkle with the walnuts. Serve immediately.

Serves 2

• Walnut Coleslaw •

Crunchy and fresh, this salad of sprouts and walnuts is a delicious twist on the more traditional recipe.

> TOTAL CARBOHYDRATES: 7.5 *grams*
>
> PER SERVING: 3.8 *grams*

½ *cup chopped cabbage*	1 *tablespoon Dijon mustard*
½ *cup alfalfa sprouts*	1 *teaspoon balsamic vinegar*
¼ *cup chopped walnuts*	*salt and pepper to taste*
¼ *cup mayonnaise*	

• **Combine the cabbage, sprouts, walnuts, mayonnaise, mustard, vinegar, salt, and pepper in a large bowl. Mix well. Serve immediately.**

Serves 2

• Celery Root Salad •

Celery root has a clean flavor and crunchy texture. It's a seasonal vegetable, not available year-round, but an equal amount of chopped celery can be substituted. Serve this salad with Spiced Skirt Steak (page 127).

> **TOTAL CARBOHYDRATES: 8.7 grams**
>
> **PER SERVING: 4.4 grams**

2 tablespoons mayonnaise
1 teaspoon Dijon mustard
2 teaspoons balsamic vinegar
salt and pepper to taste

1 cup peeled and coarsely
  chopped celery root
1 tablespoon chopped fresh
  cilantro or parsley

• **Combine the mayonnaise, mustard, vinegar, salt, pepper, and celery root in a bowl and mix well. Sprinkle with the cilantro and serve immediately.**

Serves 2

• Red Cabbage Salad with •
Feta and Dill

A friend created this colorful salad for a potluck dinner, and ever since it has been her most requested dish for informal get-togethers and picnics.

> TOTAL CARBOHYDRATES: *16.1 grams*
>
> PER SERVING: *8.1 grams*

¼ cup olive oil
juice of ½ lemon
1 clove garlic, minced
salt and pepper to taste
1½ cups chopped red cabbage

¼ cup pine nuts, lightly
    toasted (see Hint on
    page 163)
½ cup crumbled feta cheese
⅓ cup chopped fresh dill

• **Whisk together the oil, lemon juice, garlic, salt, and pepper in a large serving bowl. Add the cabbage, pine nuts, feta, and dill, and toss well. Serve immediately.**

Serves 2

• Greek Salad •

This snappy salad makes a delicious lunch or first course.

> **TOTAL CARBOHYDRATES:** *15.5 grams*
>
> **PER SERVING:** *7.8 grams*

1 medium tomato, cut into
    2-inch pieces
1 cucumber, peeled, seeded,
    and sliced
¼ cup thinly sliced red onion
⅓ cup crumbled feta cheese

2 Kalamata olives, cut into
    slivers (optional)
3 tablespoons olive oil
1 tablespoon red wine vinegar
salt and pepper to taste

• **Combine the tomato, cucumber, onion, feta, and olives, if using, in a large serving bowl. Whisk together the oil, vinegar, salt, and pepper in a small bowl. Pour the dressing over the salad and toss well. Serve immediately.**

Serves 2

· Mixed Green Salad with ·
Warm Bacon Dressing

Smoky bacon and sweet sautéed leek combine in a flavor-packed salad dressing that blends beautifully with assorted greens.

> TOTAL CARBOHYDRATES: *12.2 grams*
>
> PER SERVING: *6.1 grams*

1 ½ ounces sliced slab bacon, cut into 1-inch pieces
1 leek (white part only), halved lengthwise, washed well, and thinly sliced crosswise
3 tablespoons olive oil

1 tablespoon red wine vinegar
salt and pepper to taste
5 cups torn assorted lettuce leaves (such as Boston, romaine, and red leaf), washed and spun dry

● Sauté the bacon in a heavy skillet over medium-high heat, stirring, for about 2 to 3 minutes, until it turns golden brown. Add the leek to the skillet and sauté, stirring, for about 4 minutes. Turn the heat to medium-low. Add the oil, vinegar, salt, and pepper, and cook for 1 minute. Place the lettuce leaves in a large bowl, pour the bacon dressing over them, and toss gently. Serve immediately.

Serves 2

· Warm Spinach Salad ·
with Bacon and Pine Nuts

You'll love this variation on the traditional spinach salad. The texture of the pine nuts mellows the saltiness of the bacon and the tanginess of the vinegar.

TOTAL CARBOHYDRATES: *12.5 grams*

PER SERVING: *6.3 grams*

2 tablespoons olive oil
4 slices slab bacon, cut into
      ¹/₂-inch pieces
2 tablespoons pine nuts
2 small cloves garlic,
      minced

1 pound spinach leaves,
      trimmed, washed well,
      and spun dry
1 tablespoon balsamic vinegar
1 tablespoon grated Parmesan
      cheese

• **Heat 1 tablespoon of oil in a heavy skillet over medium-high heat until hot but not smoking. Add the bacon and sauté, stirring occasionally, for 4 minutes, or until browned. Turn the heat to medium, add the pine nuts, and cook for 1 minute, stirring occasionally. Add the garlic and cook, stirring, for 30 seconds. Add the spinach, vinegar, and remaining tablespoon of oil, cook, tossing gently, for 15 seconds, or until the spinach is warm and a bit wilted. Transfer to serving plates, sprinkle with Parmesan, and serve immediately.**

Serves 2

• Cucumber and Tomato Salad •
with Mortadella

This hearty salad with mortadella sausage has a wonderful Italian flavor, but you can use any leftover meat.

> TOTAL CARBOHYDRATES: *21.2 grams*
>
> PER SERVING: *10.6 grams*

¼ cup olive oil
2 tablespoons fresh lemon
    juice
2 tablespoons chopped fresh
    parsley
2 tablespoons chopped fresh
    dill

2 cloves garlic, minced
salt and pepper to taste
1 cup diced mortadella
    sausage
1 cup diced cucumber
⅓ cup chopped onion
1 medium tomato, diced

• **Whisk together the oil, lemon juice, parsley, dill, garlic, salt, and pepper until smooth. Combine the mortadella, cucumber, onion, and tomato in a large serving bowl. Pour the dressing over the salad, toss gently, and serve immediately.**

Serves 2

• Bacon and Cabbage Salad •

This sturdy salad is a Russian version of coleslaw. You can add leftover meat or chicken to it to create a satisfying luncheon salad.

TOTAL CARBOHYDRATES: 17.2 grams

PER SERVING: 8.6 grams

¼ pound bacon
1 cup chopped cabbage
1 half-sour pickle, chopped
½ cup sauerkraut

2 scallions (white part only),
    chopped
salt and pepper to taste

• Sauté the bacon in a heavy skillet over medium-high heat for about 5 minutes, until crispy and brown. Remove the bacon from the skillet, reserving 1 tablespoon of bacon grease, and crumble. Combine the cabbage, pickle, sauerkraut, scallions, crumbled bacon, salt, pepper, and reserved bacon grease in a bowl and toss well. Serve immediately.

Serves 2

Main Courses

•

EGGS

SEAFOOD

POULTRY

PORK

LAMB

VEAL

BEEF

Eggs

•

Poached Eggs

Mustard Scrambled Eggs

Baked Eggs in Bacon Rings

Baked Eggs with Swiss Cheese and Cream

Ricotta and Leek Frittata

Smoked Salmon Frittata

Herb Kookoo (Frittata with Herbs)

Eggs Benedict with Spinach

Egg Salad with Capers

• Poached Eggs •

Poaching is a wonderful way to prepare eggs, and poached eggs form the basis of any number of classic dishes, such as Eggs Benedict. The addition of vinegar to the water helps the egg whites hold their shape.

> TOTAL CARBOHYDRATES: *0 grams*
>
> PER SERVING: *0 grams*

2 tablespoons white vinegar
1 teaspoon salt
4 large eggs

Bring to a boil enough water to inch up the side of a large, deep skillet. Add the vinegar and salt, and bring to a bare simmer. Break the eggs, one at a time, into a saucer or small bowl and slip them into the water. Poach the eggs over low heat until the whites are firm, 2 to 3 minutes. Remove the eggs with a slotted spoon. Serve immediately.

Serves 2

• Mustard Scrambled Eggs •

Dr. Atkins loves to make breakfast on weekends, and he often comes up with some very unusual and tasty combinations. This is one of his favorites. Serve with bacon or sausage on the side.

> TOTAL CARBOHYDRATES: 2.7 grams
>
> PER SERVING: 1.4 grams

4 eggs
1 teaspoon mustard powder
1/2 teaspoon crumbled dried
    oregano

1 tablespoon hot water
2 tablespoons sour cream
2 tablespoons butter
salt and pepper to taste

• **Combine the eggs, mustard powder, oregano, water, and sour cream in a bowl and beat lightly. Heat the butter in a skillet over medium heat until the foam subsides. Add the egg mixture and cook, stirring, about 4 minutes, until the mixture becomes custardlike but not loose. Sprinkle with salt and pepper, and serve immediately.**

Serves 2

• Baked Eggs in Bacon Rings •

These baked eggs are the perfect entree for a lazy brunch with the Sunday paper.

> TOTAL CARBOHYDRATES: *7.2 grams*
>
> PER SERVING: *3.6 grams*

6 strips bacon
melted butter for brushing
    the tins
4 slices tomato, each about
    ½ inch thick

4 eggs
salt and pepper to taste
sour cream as an
    accompaniment
    (optional)

- **Preheat the oven to 325°F.**

  Cook the bacon in a skillet over medium heat until it begins to shrivel, about 3 minutes. Remove from the heat. Brush 4 cups in a muffin tin or four 5-ounce ramekins with the melted butter. Place a tomato slice in the bottom of each cup. Circle the inside of each cup with 1½ strips of bacon. Break an egg into each muffin cup and season with salt and pepper. Fill any unused tins with water to protect them from burning. Bake in the oven for 20 minutes.

  To serve, loosen the edges of the eggs with a spatula and transfer the eggs to plates. Top each egg with a dollop of sour cream if desired.

Serves 2

• Baked Eggs with Swiss Cheese • and Cream

Baked eggs, or shirred eggs, make great individual meals. This recipe calls for 10-ounce ramekins, but if you only have smaller ones, use one egg instead of two in each ramekin.

> TOTAL CARBOHYDRATES: *3.2 grams*
>
> PER SERVING: *1.6 grams*

2 tablespoons butter, softened
4 large eggs
½ cup grated Swiss cheese
½ cup heavy cream, heated

salt and pepper to taste
crumbled cooked bacon for garnish

- **Preheat the oven to 350°F.**

Butter 2 large (10-ounce) ramekins and break 2 eggs into each one. Cover each portion with half the cheese and half the heated cream, and season with salt and pepper.

Place the ramekins in a pan filled with enough water to come halfway up the sides of the ramekins. Bake in the oven for 15 minutes, or until the cheese has melted and the egg whites are mostly firm. Remove the ramekins from the oven and preheat the broiler. Place the ramekins under the broiler for 2 to 3 minutes, or until the cheese begins to brown. Serve immediately with the crumbled bacon on top.

Serves 2

• Ricotta and Leek Frittata •

Leeks become marvelously sweet when they are sautéed. Here, they give an extra measure of flavor to this frittata. Serve with a mixed green salad.

> TOTAL CARBOHYDRATES: 3.9 grams
>
> PER SERVING: 2 grams

1 tablespoon butter
1 leek (white part only),
    halved lengthwise,
    washed well, and cut
    into ½-inch pieces

1½ tablespoons whole-milk
    ricotta cheese
salt and pepper to taste
4 eggs, lightly beaten

• **Preheat the broiler.**

Heat half of the butter in a 10-inch flameproof skillet (preferably nonstick) over medium-high heat until the foam subsides. Add the leek and sauté, stirring, for 3 minutes. Remove from the heat and cool.

Add the sautéed leek, ricotta, salt, and pepper to the beaten eggs and mix well. Heat the remaining butter in the skillet over medium heat until the foam subsides. Pour in the egg mixture and cook, stirring, about 1 minute, until the egg starts to form curds. Cook for another minute (the egg mixture should be set on the bottom and still a bit wet on top).

Place the skillet under the broiler for about 2 minutes, until the frittata turns golden brown. Using a spatula, carefully remove the frittata from the skillet. Cut into wedges and serve.

Serves 2

• Smoked Salmon Frittata •

Eggs are not just for breakfast. This elegant frittata is perfect for a late supper. For special occasions, serve it with sour cream and caviar.

> TOTAL CARBOHYDRATES: .5 gram
>
> PER SERVING: .3 gram

4 large eggs, lightly beaten
1 ounce smoked salmon,
     chopped
1 teaspoon chopped fresh
     chives

1 tablespoon sour cream
salt and pepper to taste
1 tablespoon butter

- **Preheat the broiler.**

Beat together the eggs, salmon, chives, sour cream, salt, and pepper in a bowl. Heat the butter in a 10-inch flameproof skillet (preferably nonstick) over medium heat until the foam subsides. Pour in the egg mixture and cook, stirring, about 1 minute, until the egg starts to form curds. Cook for another minute (the egg mixture should be set on the bottom and still a bit wet on top).

Place the skillet under the broiler and broil about 2 minutes, until the frittata turns golden brown. Using a spatula, carefully remove the frittata from the skillet. Cut into wedges and serve.

Serves 2

• Herb Kookoo •
(Frittata with Herbs)

No doubt about it, we are absolutely cuckoo for this Middle Eastern version of a frittata that we adapted from *Food of Life* by Najmieh Batmanglij. Kookoos and frittatas are usually served at room temperature, cut into wedges. When accompanied by a great salad, the dish makes a main course. For a variation, try using a slice of kookoo as the "base" for an open-faced, knife-and-fork sandwich of ham and Swiss cheese or chicken salad. Experiment with your own favorite flavor combinations. You usually can't go wrong with a kookoo.

> TOTAL CARBOHYDRATES: *14.2 grams*
> PER SERVING: *7.1 grams*

½ cup chopped scallion (white part only)
1 cup chopped fresh flat-leaf parsley
½ cup chopped fresh dill
½ cup chopped fresh cilantro

8 large eggs
¼ teaspoon freshly ground pepper
½ teaspoon baking soda
1 teaspoon salt
¼ cup olive or canola oil

• Combine the scallion, parsley, dill, and cilantro in a food processor and blend for 5 seconds. Scrape down the side and add the eggs, pepper, baking soda, salt, and 2 tablespoons of the oil. Blend the mixture for about 30 seconds, or until smooth.

Heat the remaining oil in a heavy skillet over medium heat until hot but not smoking. Add the egg mixture to the skillet, cover, and cook it over low heat for about 15 minutes, stirring once during the first 7 minutes or until it is set. Cut the kookoo into 4 wedges and turn the wedges 1 at a time. Cook the kookoo for another 5 minutes. Remove from the pan and let cool for 2 minutes. Serve immediately or store in the refrigerator for up to 2 days.

Serves 2

• Eggs Benedict with Spinach •

Eggs Benedict and Eggs Florentine combine in this savory dish.
Serve as a lunch or brunch entree.

> TOTAL CARBOHYDRATES: 5.4 grams
>
> PER SERVING: 2.7 grams

4 pieces Canadian bacon
1 cup thawed and cooked
   frozen or fresh spinach
4 Poached Eggs (page 64)
¼ cup Quick and Easy
   Hollandaise Sauce (page
   171)

2 teaspoons chopped fresh
   flat-leaf parsley or dill
   for garnish (optional)

● Heat a skillet over medium heat until hot but not smoking.
Add the Canadian bacon and cook about 2 minutes on each side,
until lightly browned. Divide the spinach between 2 plates. Top
each serving with 2 pieces of bacon and 2 poached eggs. Spoon
the Hollandaise over the eggs and sprinkle with parsley if desired. Serve immediately.

Serves 2

Variation: For a different taste, substitute 2 thin slices of
smoked salmon for the Canadian bacon.

• Egg Salad with Capers •

You can't go wrong with this egg salad for a quick lunch. It is served on a bed of crisp lettuce.

TOTAL CARBOHYDRATES: *2.2 grams*
PER SERVING: *1.1 grams*

4 hard-boiled eggs, peeled and
    chopped
2 tablespoons mayonnaise
1 teaspoon Dijon mustard
2 tablespoons chopped celery
1 tablespoon small capers or
    chopped large capers

½ teaspoon chopped fresh
    tarragon or ¼ teaspoon
    crumbled dried tarragon
salt and pepper to taste

• **Combine the eggs, mayonnaise, mustard, celery, capers, tarragon, salt, and pepper in a bowl and mix well. Serve or store, covered, in the refrigerator for up to 1 day.**

Serves 2

Seafood

•

Scallops with Thyme

Scallops in Sherry-Cream Sauce

Stir-Fried Shrimp with Ginger and Mushrooms

Shrimp Scampi

Tarragon Shrimp Salad

Sautéed Sole

Sautéed Cod with Lemon-Parsley Sauce

Red Snapper with Tomato and Olives

Oven-Poached Salmon with Dill and Wine

Salmon Burgers

Tuna with Ginger and Soy

Peppers Stuffed with Walnut Tuna Salad

Pepper-Crusted Swordfish

Squid with Basil and Lime

Sautéed Soft-Shell Crabs

Crab and Avocado Salad

• Scallops with Thyme •

The rich, succulent flavor of scallops is complemented here by the tangy lemon and fresh thyme. Serve with Orange Daikon Salad (page 49).

> TOTAL CARBOHYDRATES: 18.5 grams
>
> PER SERVING: 9.3 grams

2 teaspoons salt
1 teaspoon cayenne pepper
1 pound sea scallops, rinsed
  and patted dry
3 tablespoons butter
2 cloves garlic, minced

2 scallions (white part only),
  chopped
1 tablespoon fresh thyme or
  1½ teaspoons crumbled
  dried thyme
juice of ½ lemon

• **Combine the salt and cayenne in a small bowl. Sprinkle the mixture over the scallops. Heat the butter in a heavy skillet or a wok over medium-high heat until it is bubbling and beginning to brown. Add the garlic and scallions, and cook, stirring, for 30 seconds. Add the scallops and thyme to the skillet and cook, turning the scallops, about 4 minutes, until they are lightly browned. Drizzle with the lemon juice and serve immediately.**

Serves 2

• Scallops in Sherry-Cream Sauce •

These elegant scallops have a distinct French flavor. Serve with Cauliflower and Mushroom Puree (140) or steamed green beans for a perfect supper.

> TOTAL CARBOHYDRATES: *18.5 grams*
> PER SERVING: *9.5 grams*

2 tablespoons butter
1 pound bay scallops, rinsed
    and patted dry
2 tablespoons minced shallots
1/2 cup sliced mushrooms

1/3 cup dry sherry
2 egg yolks
1/2 cup heavy cream
salt and pepper to taste

• Heat 1 tablespoon of the butter in a large, heavy skillet over medium-high heat until the foam subsides. Add the scallops and sauté, stirring occasionally, for 3 to 4 minutes, or until opaque and slightly firm. Remove from the skillet and keep warm.

Heat the remaining tablespoon of butter in the skillet until the foam subsides. Add the shallots and mushrooms, and sauté for 2 minutes, stirring occasionally. Add the sherry and bring to a boil. Lower the heat and simmer for 3 minutes, making sure to scrape up any brown bits from the bottom of the skillet.

Whisk together the egg yolks and cream in a small bowl. Gradually whisk the egg mixture into the mushroom mixture, and add the salt and pepper. Return the scallops to the skillet and coat well with the sauce. Serve immediately.

Serves 2

· Stir-Fried Shrimp with · Ginger and Mushrooms

A quick and easy stir-fry is a perfect weekday supper. In this recipe you can substitute for the shrimp an equal amount of chicken breast, cut into strips.

> TOTAL CARBOHYDRATES: *10.7 grams*
>
> PER SERVING: *5.4 grams*

1 tablespoon canola oil
2 cloves garlic, minced
1 tablespoon peeled and
    chopped gingerroot
½ cup sliced mushrooms
½ cup chopped celery
1 tablespoon toasted sesame
    oil

1 tablespoon soy sauce
¼ teaspoon dried hot red
    pepper flakes, or to taste
¾ pound shrimp, shelled and
    deveined

• Heat the canola oil in a large, heavy skillet or a wok over medium-high heat until hot but not smoking. Add the garlic and gingerroot, and stir-fry for 30 seconds. Add the mushrooms, celery, sesame oil, soy sauce, red pepper flakes, and shrimp. Stir-fry until the shrimp are pink and just cooked through, 3 to 4 minutes. Serve immediately.

Serves 2

• Shrimp Scampi •

Lemon, wine, and garlic do wonders for shrimp. This dish is very easy to make and is always a hit. You can easily double the recipe to serve guests.

> TOTAL CARBOHYDRATES: *13.2 grams*
>
> PER SERVING: *6.6 grams*

2 tablespoons butter
2 tablespoons olive oil
4 large cloves garlic, minced
1/4 cup chopped fresh flat-leaf
    parsley
juice of 1/2 lemon

1/2 cup dry white wine
pinch of dried hot red pepper
    flakes
salt and black pepper to taste
1 pound large shrimp, shelled
    and deveined

• Heat the butter and oil in a heavy skillet over medium heat until the foam subsides. Add the garlic, parsley, lemon juice, wine, pepper flakes, salt, and pepper. Bring to a boil, lower the heat, and simmer for 3 minutes. Add the shrimp to the skillet and cook, stirring frequently, for 5 to 6 minutes, until the shrimp are pink. Remove from the heat. Place the shrimp on a serving plate and pour the sauce from the skillet over them. Serve immediately.

Serves 2

· Tarragon Shrimp Salad ·

Cool and refreshing, this tarragon-infused shrimp salad is a perfect light luncheon. Serve it on a bed of crisp mixed greens.

> TOTAL CARBOHYDRATES: *7.6 grams*
>
> PER SERVING: *3.8 grams*

½ cup mayonnaise
2 tablespoons Dijon mustard
½ teaspoon Anchovy Paste
    (page 159) or 1 oil-
    packed anchovy fillet,
    mashed
½ tablespoon small capers or
    chopped large capers
½ tablespoon chopped fresh
    flat-leaf parsley

½ tablespoon chopped fresh
    tarragon or ¾ teaspoon
    crumbled dried tarragon
salt and pepper to taste
¾ pound cooked medium
    shrimp, shelled and
    deveined

● **Whisk together the mayonnaise, mustard, anchovy paste, capers, parsley, tarragon, salt, and pepper in a large serving bowl. Add the shrimp and toss the salad well. Serve immediately.**

Serves 2

• Sautéed Sole •

This crispy sole is especially good when served with Caper Tartar Sauce (page 169) or Sorrel Sauce (page 157).

> TOTAL CARBOHYDRATES:
>
> with Breading I (Pork Rind–Sesame Breading): 1.8 grams
>
> with Breading II (Sesame-Tofu Breading): 5.6 grams
>
> with Breading III (Pork Rind–Tofu Breading): 1.9 grams
>
> PER SERVING:
>
> with Breading I: .9 gram
>
> with Breading II: 2.8 grams
>
> with Breading III: .9 gram

1½ pounds sole fillets
salt and pepper to taste
1 egg, lightly beaten
¼ cup breading (I, II, or III;
    see pages 190–192)

2 tablespoons butter
2 tablespoons olive oil

• Season the sole fillets with salt and pepper. Dip the fillets in the egg and dredge in the breading, shaking off any excess. Heat the butter and oil in a large skillet over medium-high heat until the foam subsides. Sauté the sole, in batches if necessary (do not crowd the skillet), for 2 minutes on each side. Drain the fillets on paper towels and serve immediately.

Serves 2

· Sautéed Cod with ·
Lemon-Parsley Sauce

Cod has a very delicate flavor and texture, so it tends to fall apart when sautéed. Don't worry about a less-than-perfect presentation—the taste makes up for it.

> TOTAL CARBOHYDRATES: *6.6 grams*
>
> PER SERVING: *3.3 grams*

1 tablespoon butter	1½ tablespoons chopped fresh
1 tablespoon olive oil	flat-leaf parsley
3 cloves garlic, thinly sliced	1 tablespoon fresh thyme or
½ cup chopped onion	1½ teaspoons crumbled
1 pound cod fillets	dried thyme
juice of ½ lemon	salt and pepper to taste

● Heat the butter and oil in a skillet over medium-high heat until the foam subsides. Add the garlic and sauté, stirring, for 5 seconds. Add the onion and sauté for 1 minute. Add the cod and sauté for 5 minutes, turning once (the fish will crumble). Add the lemon juice, parsley, thyme, salt, and pepper. Cover the skillet and cook the fish about 2 minutes, until the cod is opaque and flaky. Serve immediately.

Serves 2

• Red Snapper with Tomato •
and Olives

The lusty flavors of classic Italian *puttanesca* sauce—tomatoes, capers, black olives—have a wonderful affinity for firm-fleshed red snapper. Serve with Wax Beans with Garlic-Tarragon Vinaigrette (page 143).

> TOTAL CARBOHYDRATES: *16.3 grams*
>
> PER SERVING: *8.2 grams*

1 tablespoon olive oil
½ small onion, chopped
1 clove garlic, minced
5 Greek black olives, pitted
    and chopped
¾ cup chopped tomatoes

2 tablespoons capers
¼ cup dry red wine
pinch of dried hot red pepper
    flakes (optional)
2 tablespoons butter
1½ pounds red snapper fillets

• Heat the oil in a large skillet over medium heat until hot but not smoking. Add the onion, garlic, and olives. Cook, stirring occasionally, for 3 minutes, or until the onion is transparent. Add the tomatoes, capers, wine, and red pepper flakes, if using. Bring to a boil, lower the heat, and simmer for 5 minutes.

Meanwhile, heat the butter in another large skillet over medium heat until the foam subsides. Cook the snapper for 2 minutes on each side, or until lightly browned. Transfer the snapper to the tomato mixture in the skillet, cover, and cook over medium heat for 3 minutes, or until the snapper just flakes. Serve immediately.

Serves 2

· Oven-Poached Salmon with ·
Dill and Wine

Fresh salmon has a very delicate flavor, and oven-poaching will keep it moist and tasty. Serve the salmon warm with lemon wedges or chilled with Cucumber-Dill Sauce (page 166), Creamy Celery Sauce (page 167), or Horseradish Cream (page 168).

TOTAL CARBOHYDRATES: 4.6 grams

PER SERVING: 2.3 grams

1 pound salmon steak (about 1 inch thick)
salt and pepper to taste
3 tablespoons chopped fresh dill

3 tablespoons fresh lemon or lime juice
3 tablespoons dry white wine
1 bay leaf

• **Preheat the oven to 375°F. Place the salmon steak on 2 layers of aluminum foil, twice as big as the salmon. Salt and pepper the salmon. Bring up all sides of the foil and carefully add the dill, lemon juice, wine, and bay leaf. Fold all sides of the foil together, creating a tent over the salmon.**

Place the salmon tent on a baking sheet and bake for 20 minutes. Remove from the oven and carefully unwrap the top of the foil (the steam will be very hot). Gently transfer the salmon to a serving plate, discarding the bay leaf. Pour any liquid in the foil over the fish. Serve immediately.

Serves 2

• Salmon Burgers •

Here's a great alternative to beef burgers, and you'll probably have all the ingredients you need in your pantry. Serve with Cilantro-Lime Pesto (page 161) or Cucumber-Dill Sauce (page 166).

TOTAL CARBOHYDRATES:

with Breading I (Pork Rind–Sesame Breading): 9.1 grams

with Breading II (Sesame-Tofu Breading): 15.2 grams

with Breading III (Pork Rind–Tofu Breading): 9.1 grams

PER SERVING:

with Breading I: 4.6 grams

with Breading II: 7.6 grams

with Breading III: 4.6 grams

one 12-ounce can salmon
1/2 cup finely chopped onion
3 tablespoons chopped fresh
    dill
2 large eggs
1/3 cup breading (I, II, or III;
    see pages 190–192)

dash of hot pepper sauce
    (optional)
salt and pepper to taste
2 tablespoons butter
1 tablespoon vegetable oil

• Combine the salmon, onion, dill, eggs, breading, hot pepper sauce, if using, salt, and pepper in a bowl and mix well. Form into 2 patties, each about 3 inches in diameter. Heat the butter and oil in a heavy skillet over medium-high heat until the foam subsides. Sauté the salmon patties, turning them once, for 3 to 4 minutes, until golden. Serve immediately.

Serves 2

• Tuna with Ginger and Soy •

The Asian flavors of gingerroot and soy make this tuna fragrant and delicious. If you do not have a grill, you can pan-sear the tuna over medium-high heat for four minutes on each side.

> TOTAL CARBOHYDRATES: 5.9 *grams*
>
> PER SERVING: *3 grams*

1 pound fresh tuna (about 2 inches thick), cut into 2 steaks
3 tablespoons soy sauce
⅓ cup olive oil

½ cup white wine
1 tablespoon chopped fresh gingerroot
3 tablespoons heavy cream

- **Preheat the grill.**

Place the tuna in a ceramic or glass bowl. In another bowl, whisk together the soy sauce, oil, wine, and gingerroot. Pour the mixture over the tuna and let the tuna marinate, covered, in the refrigerator for 15 minutes, turning it once. Remove the tuna from the marinade, pat it dry, and grill it for 4 minutes on each side.

While the tuna is grilling, pour the marinade into a saucepan, bring to a boil, and boil for 5 minutes. Lower the heat, add the cream, and simmer the sauce for 1 minute (do not let it boil). Transfer the tuna to plates and pour the sauce over it. Serve immediately.

Serves 2

Peppers Stuffed with
Walnut Tuna Salad

You'll never miss the bread with this zesty version of a quick tuna salad. For a more hearty winter lunch, add grated cheese to the top and bake for a few minutes. It makes a great tuna melt.

> TOTAL CARBOHYDRATES: 16.9 grams
>
> PER SERVING: 8.5 grams

one 6-ounce can chunk white
   tuna, drained
$1/4$ cup chopped walnuts
$1/2$ cup chopped scallion (white
   part only)
juice of $1/2$ lemon
1 teaspoon olive oil
2 tablespoons mayonnaise
$1/2$ teaspoon Dijon mustard

$1/4$ teaspoon white pepper
salt to taste
1 bell pepper, cut in half and
   seeded
1 tablespoon chopped fresh
   dill (optional)
2 thin lemon slices for garnish
   (optional)

● **Combine the tuna, walnuts, scallion, lemon juice, oil, mayonnaise, mustard, white pepper, and salt in a bowl and mix well. Fill each pepper half with half the tuna mixture. Sprinkle with the dill and garnish with the lemon slices if desired. Serve immediately.**

Serves 2

• *Pepper-Crusted Swordfish* •

Meaty, rich swordfish makes a perfect foil for this spicy, aromatic crust. Serve with Cucumber in Cream Sauce (page 141).

TOTAL CARBOHYDRATES: *8.8 grams*
PER SERVING: *4.4 grams*

¾ pound swordfish steak
(about 1 inch thick), cut
into 2 pieces
juice of ½ lime
1 tablespoon coarsely ground
coriander seeds

2 tablespoons coarsely ground
black peppercorns
¼ cup coarsely ground
hazelnuts
salt to taste
2 tablespoons butter, softened

- **Preheat the broiler.**
  Drizzle the swordfish with the lime juice and broil for 3 minutes on each side. Meanwhile, combine the coriander, peppercorns, hazelnuts, and salt in a bowl and mix well. Let the swordfish cool slightly. Pat the peppercorn mixture on all sides of the fish and dot with the butter. Broil the swordfish for 4 minutes, turning once. Serve immediately.

Serves 2

• Squid with Basil and Lime •

Sweet basil blends beautifully with the mild, almost nutty flavor of squid. Squid freezes well, so if you don't have access to fresh squid, the frozen product is fine. Serve with mixed baby greens.

TOTAL CARBOHYDRATES: *18.7 grams*	
PER SERVING: *9.4 grams*	

1 pound cleaned squid, bodies
  cut into ½-inch rings
  and tentacles halved
½ cup chopped fresh basil
  leaves
2 tablespoons olive oil

juice of 1 lime
1 clove garlic, minced
¼ teaspoon dried hot red
  pepper flakes
1 tablespoon peanut oil

• Combine the squid, basil, olive oil, lime juice, garlic, and red pepper flakes in a bowl and mix well. Let the squid marinate, covered, in the refrigerator for at least 20 minutes and up to 1 hour.

Heat a wok or heavy skillet over medium-high heat until a drop of water sizzles on the surface, about 45 seconds. Pour the peanut oil into the wok, add the squid, and cook, stirring frequently, about 4 minutes, until the squid is opaque and tender. Serve immediately.

Serves 2

Variation: You can easily adapt this recipe to create a delightful seafood salad. Chill the Squid with Basil and Lime for 30 minutes. Add ½ cup each of chopped celery and chopped bell pepper. Whisk together 3 tablespoons of oil and 1 tablespoon of fresh lemon juice. Drizzle the dressing over the salad, toss gently, and serve.

• Sautéed Soft-Shell Crabs •

Crispy and delicious, these soft-shell crabs need only a drizzling of lemon juice and a dollop of Caper Tartar Sauce (page 169) to make a succulent seafood entree.

> TOTAL CARBOHYDRATES: *8.5 grams*
>
> PER SERVING: *1.4 grams per prepared crab*

2 tablespoons tofu or soy flour
    (available at natural-
    food stores)
2 tablespoons ground
    hazelnuts

salt and pepper to taste
6 cleaned soft-shell crabs,
    washed and patted dry
1 tablespoon butter
1 tablespoon olive oil

• Stir together the tofu flour, ground hazelnuts, salt, and pepper on a large plate. Dredge the crabs in this flour mixture, shaking off any excess.

Heat the butter and oil in a large, heavy skillet over medium-high heat until the foam subsides. Sauté the crabs for 4 to 5 minutes on each side, or until lightly browned. Drain on paper towels and serve immediately.

Serves 2 or 3

• Crab and Avocado Salad •

Sweet crabmeat and creamy avocado combine in this delectable salad with a spicy fragrance.

TOTAL CARBOHYDRATES: 12.1 grams

PER SERVING: 6.1 grams

$\frac{1}{3}$ cup chopped celery

$\frac{1}{2}$ pound cooked fresh crabmeat; or frozen crabmeat, thawed, or canned crabmeat, drained

1 tablespoon mayonnaise

1 teaspoon cumin

$\frac{1}{2}$ teaspoon turmeric

1 tablespoon capers

salt and pepper to taste

juice of $\frac{1}{2}$ lemon

$\frac{1}{2}$ medium Haas avocado, cubed and drizzled with lemon juice

1 bunch watercress, stems removed

● **Combine the celery, crabmeat, mayonnaise, cumin, turmeric, capers, salt, pepper, and lemon juice in a large bowl and mix well. Gently stir in the avocado. Divide the watercress between 2 plates, top with the crab salad, and serve immediately.**

Serves 2

Poultry

•

Chicken Cutlets
Chicken with Lemon and Capers
Coconut Chicken Satés with Cilantro
Chicken with Coconut-Plum Sauce
Chicken with Cucumber
Chicken with Indian Spices
Chicken Paprika
Creamed Chicken with Mushrooms
Chicken Salad with Pesto and Fennel
Curried Chicken Salad with Cucumber
Fried Chicken Salad with Stilton
Cornish Game Hens with White Wine Sauce
Breast of Duck with Red Wine Sauce

• Chicken Cutlets •

Chicken cutlets are a quick and easy staple of home cooking. Serve the following version in the traditional manner with a drizzling of lemon juice, or cut the chicken into julienne strips and serve with Warm Spinach Salad with Bacon and Pine Nuts (page 57).

TOTAL CARBOHYDRATES:

with Breading I (Pork Rind–Sesame Breading): 1.8 grams

with Breading II (Sesame-Tofu Breading): 5.6 grams

with Breading III (Pork Rind–Tofu Breading): 1.9 grams

PER SERVING:

with Breading I: .9 gram

with Breading II: 2.8 grams

with Breading III: .9 gram

2 whole boneless chicken breasts, halved
1 egg, lightly beaten
1/3 cup breading (I, II, or III; pages 190–192)

2 tablespoons olive or canola oil
2 tablespoons butter
1 tablespoon chopped parsley for garnish

• Dip each chicken breast into the egg and then into the breading, making sure the chicken is coated by the breading. Shake off any excess.

Heat the oil and butter in a heavy skillet over medium heat until hot but not smoking. Add and cook the chicken, in batches if necessary, for 4 minutes per side, until golden brown. Remove the chicken breasts to a platter, sprinkle with parsley, and serve immediately.

Serves 2

• Chicken with Lemon and Capers •

Tangy capers are a natural partner for chicken. In this dish the capers and lemon juice are mellowed when butter is whisked into the liquid, creating a rich sauce.

> TOTAL CARBOHYDRATES: *2.8 grams*
>
> PER SERVING: *1.4 grams*

1 tablespoon olive oil
2 whole boneless chicken
    breasts, halved
1/3 cup white wine
1 tablespoon lemon juice

1 teaspoon grated lemon zest
1 tablespoon capers
2 tablespoons chilled butter,
    cut into small pieces

• Heat the oil in a heavy skillet over medium heat until hot but not smoking. Add the chicken and cook for 4 minutes on each side, or until browned. Remove the chicken from the skillet and keep warm.

Add the wine, lemon juice, lemon zest, and capers to the skillet. Bring to a boil, lower the heat, and simmer for 2 minutes, making sure to scrape up any brown bits from the bottom of the skillet. Whisk in the butter, 1 piece at a time, and cook over low heat for 1 minute, or until heated through. Pour the sauce over the chicken and serve immediately.

Serves 2

• Coconut Chicken Satés •
with Cilantro

The coconut milk marinade makes these chicken satés, a popular Thai dish, tender and juicy. Peanut Dipping Sauce (page 165) is the traditional accompaniment.

> TOTAL CARBOHYDRATES: *6.9 grams*
>
> PER SERVING: *3.5 grams*

one 14-ounce can unsweetened coconut milk; reserve 1 tablespoon if making the Peanut Dipping Sauce
⅓ cup chopped fresh cilantro
1 teaspoon chopped fresh jalapeño pepper
1 small clove garlic, minced
juice of ½ lime
salt and pepper to taste
2 whole boneless chicken breasts, cut into 1-inch strips
10 bamboo skewers, soaked in water for 30 minutes, or 10 metal skewers (see Note)

● **Preheat the broiler.**

Combine the coconut milk, cilantro, jalapeño, garlic, lime juice, salt, and pepper in a large bowl and mix well. Add the chicken, stirring to coat. Let the chicken marinate, covered, in the refrigerator for at least 20 minutes or up to 1 hour.

Thread 2 pieces of chicken onto each skewer and broil, turning once, for 7 minutes, or until the chicken is lightly browned. Transfer to a serving plate and serve immediately.

Serves 2

Note: This dish can also be prepared without the skewers. Simply transfer the marinated strips to a broiler pan and broil in the same manner.

· Chicken with ·
Coconut-Plum Sauce

This lovely chicken dish features an unusual combination of flavors. You can double or triple the recipe for a great dinner party entree.

> TOTAL CARBOHYDRATES: *19.2 grams*
>
> PER SERVING: *9.6 grams*

2 tablespoons butter
2 whole boneless chicken
    breasts, halved
1 cup unsweetened coconut
    milk
1 tablespoon Dijon mustard
1 teaspoon crumbled dried
    tarragon or 2 teaspoons
    chopped fresh tarragon

salt and pepper to taste
1 small plum, halved, pitted,
    and thinly sliced
3 tablespoons coarsely chopped
    almonds, lightly toasted
    (see Hint on page 163)

• **Heat the butter in a large, deep skillet over medium-high heat until the foam subsides. Add the chicken and sauté about 3 minutes on each side, until lightly browned. Add the coconut milk to the skillet. Bring to a gentle boil, lower the heat, and simmer for 6 minutes, turning the chicken several times. Stir in the mustard, tarragon, salt, pepper, and sliced plum, making sure to coat the chicken, and cook over medium heat for 3 minutes. Remove from the heat and stir in the almonds. Serve immediately.**

Serves 2

• Chicken with Cucumber •

This lightly spiced chicken has a subtle flavor that makes it especially pleasing as a warm-weather meal.

> TOTAL CARBOHYDRATES: *7.9 grams*
>
> PER SERVING: *4 grams*

2 tablespoons olive oil
1 tablespoon butter
4 boneless chicken thighs, halved
1 medium cucumber, peeled, seeded, and chopped
$\frac{1}{2}$ teaspoon ground cumin
salt and pepper to taste
1 clove garlic, minced
$\frac{1}{2}$ cup chicken stock
3 tablespoons sour cream

• Heat the oil and butter in a skillet over medium heat until the foam subsides. Add the chicken and cook, turning frequently, about 10 minutes, until golden. Remove the chicken from the skillet.

Add the cucumber, cumin, salt, pepper, and garlic to the skillet and cook, stirring frequently, for 2 minutes. Return the chicken to the skillet and add the chicken stock. Bring to a boil, lower the heat, and simmer for 5 minutes. Remove from the heat and stir in the sour cream. Serve immediately.

Serves 2

• Chicken with Indian Spices •

When simmered in turmeric, also known as Indian saffron, chicken breasts become wonderfully aromatic. Turmeric has been revered for centuries, not only for its flavor but also for its medicinal properties. Rich in potassium and vitamin C, turmeric acts as an excellent anti-inflammatory, according to traditional Indian medicine. The addition of sour cream makes this dish smooth and sumptuous.

> TOTAL CARBOHYDRATES: *12.4 grams*
>
> PER SERVING: *6.2 grams*

3 tablespoons butter
1 whole boneless chicken
    breast, cut into strips
1½ teaspoons cumin
1½ teaspoons turmeric
¼ teaspoon dried hot pepper
    flakes (optional)

4 cloves garlic, minced
½ cup chicken stock
½ cup sour cream
1 tablespoon chopped fresh
    cilantro or flat-leaf
    parsley for garnish
    (optional)

• Heat the butter in a heavy casserole over medium-high heat until the foam subsides. Add the chicken strips and sauté, stirring, about 2 minutes, until browned. Add the cumin, turmeric, hot pepper flakes, and garlic, and sauté the mixture, stirring occasionally, for 2 minutes. Add the chicken stock and bring to a boil. Lower the heat to medium-low and simmer the mixture, stirring occasionally, for 10 minutes. Slowly add the sour cream and simmer the mixture (do not let it boil) for 3 minutes, or until heated through. Transfer the chicken with the sauce to a serving plate, garnish with the cilantro or parsley if desired, and serve immediately.

Serves 2

• Chicken Paprika •

The first time I made this dish, Dr. Atkins was effusive in his praise. I hope you will receive the same kudos when you serve it.

> TOTAL CARBOHYDRATES: 20.4 grams
> PER SERVING: 10.2–5.1 grams

2 tablespoons butter
¼ cup olive oil
1 cup chopped onion
1 chicken (about 3 pounds),
    cut into 8 to 12 pieces
1 tablespoon Hungarian
    paprika (available at
    specialty-food stores)

salt and pepper to taste
¼ cup chicken stock
¼ cup white wine
1 large egg yolk
½ cup sour cream

• Heat the butter and 2 tablespoons of oil in a skillet over medium-high heat until the foam subsides. Add the onion and sauté, stirring, for 3 minutes. Add the chicken pieces, skin side down, and sauté for 5 minutes on each side. Stir in the paprika, salt, pepper, and the remaining 2 tablespoons of olive oil. Cook, stirring, for about 2 minutes.

Meanwhile, bring the chicken stock and wine to a boil in a small saucepan. Whisk together the egg yolk and sour cream in a bowl. Slowly add the wine-stock mixture into the egg mixture, whisking until the sauce is smooth. Pour the sauce over the chicken in the skillet, cover, and simmer for 10 minutes. Serve immediately.

Serves 2–4

• Creamed Chicken with •
Mushrooms

A comforting food for cold nights, this creamed chicken is so good on its own that you'll never miss the traditional toast accompaniment. Just use your soup spoon to savor every last bite.

> TOTAL CARBOHYDRATES: *11.6 grams*
>
> PER SERVING: *5.8 grams*

1 whole boneless chicken
    breast, cut into 1-inch
    pieces
1 teaspoon fresh thyme or ½
    teaspoon crumbled dried
    thyme
salt and pepper to taste
3 tablespoons butter

1 cup sliced mushrooms
2 tablespoons minced shallots
⅓ cup dry white wine
⅓ cup chicken stock
½ cup heavy cream
2 tablespoons chopped fresh
    flat-leaf parsley

•   Season the chicken with the thyme, salt, and pepper. Heat 2 tablespoons of the butter in a skillet over medium-high heat until the foam subsides. Add the chicken and sauté about 3 minutes, until light golden. Add the mushrooms, stirring occasionally, for 2 minutes. Remove the chicken-mushroom mixture from the skillet and reserve.

Add the remaining tablespoon of butter to the skillet and sauté the shallots, stirring occasionally, for 2 minutes. Add the wine and stock to the skillet. Bring to a boil, lower the heat, and simmer for 5 minutes, making sure to scrape up any brown bits from the bottom of the skillet. Add the cream and gently simmer for another 5 minutes. Return the reserved chicken-mushroom mixture to the skillet, add the parsley, and cook over medium heat for 2 minutes, or until heated through. Serve immediately.

Serves 2

• Chicken Salad with Pesto • and Fennel

Fresh-tasting pesto and the licoricelike flavor of fennel permeates this delicious and unusual chicken salad.

> TOTAL CARBOHYDRATES: *9 grams*
>
> PER SERVING: *4.5 grams*

1 tablespoon butter
2 whole boneless chicken
    breasts, cut into 1-inch
    strips
juice of ½ lemon
3 tablespoons Basil Pesto (page
    160)

1 small fennel bulb, halved
    lengthwise, cored, and
    thinly sliced
½ cup chopped red bell pepper
salt and pepper to taste

• Heat the butter in a skillet over medium-high heat until the foam subsides. Add the chicken, drizzle it with the lemon juice, and sauté, turning frequently, about 5 minutes, until golden. Stir in 2 tablespoons of pesto, coating the chicken well.

Transfer the chicken to a large serving bowl. Add the fennel, red pepper, salt, pepper, and remaining pesto, and toss the salad well. Serve immediately or store, covered, in the refrigerator for up to 1 day.

Serves 2

• Curried Chicken Salad •
with Cucumber

The sweet and spicy flavor of curry powder contrasts with the coolness of cucumber in this aromatic salad. A touch of cinnamon adds a hint of intrigue.

> TOTAL CARBOHYDRATES: *8.3 grams*
>
> PER SERVING: *4.2 grams*

½ cup mayonnaise
1 teaspoon curry powder
½ teaspoon cinnamon
1 tablespoon grated onion
1 tablespoon chopped fresh
    flat-leaf parsley

1 teaspoon balsamic vinegar
salt and pepper to taste
2 cups cubed cooked chicken
½ cup chopped celery
½ cup chopped, seeded, and
    peeled cucumber

• **Whisk together the mayonnaise, curry powder, cinnamon, onion, parsley, vinegar, salt, and pepper in a large serving bowl. Add the chicken, celery, and cucumber, and toss the salad well. Serve immediately or store, covered, in the refrigerator for up to 1 day.**

Serves 2

• Fried Chicken Salad with Stilton •

Mellow blue-veined Stilton cheese and crispy fried chicken pair up to create an unbeatable flavor combination. Drizzle with Mustard Walnut Vinaigrette (page 177) or Shallot Orange Vinaigrette (page 176).

> TOTAL CARBOHYDRATES:
>
> with Breading I (Pork Rind–Sesame Breading): 11.8 grams
>
> with Breading II (Sesame-Tofu Breading): 15.6 grams
>
> with Breading III (Pork Rind–Tofu Breading): 11.9 grams
>
> PER SERVING:
>
> with Breading I: 5.9 grams
>
> with Breading II: 7.8 grams
>
> with Breading III: 6 grams

1 small head romaine lettuce, washed, torn into bite-size pieces, and spun dry
1/2 cup crumbled Stilton cheese
3 scallions (white part only), chopped
1/4 cup canola oil
1 whole boneless chicken breast, cut lengthwise into 6 strips
1 large egg, lightly beaten
1/4 cup breading (I, II, or III; pages 190–192)

• Divide the lettuce between 2 serving plates. Top each serving with half of the Stilton and half of the scallions.

Heat the oil in a heavy skillet over medium heat until hot but not smoking. Dip the chicken strips into the egg and then dredge in the breading. Shake off any excess. Fry the chicken about 5 minutes, until golden brown. Transfer the chicken to paper towels and let drain for about 1 minute. Cut the chicken into bite-size pieces and divide it between the salad plates. Serve drizzled with vinaigrette.

Serves 2

• Cornish Game Hens with •
White Wine Sauce

As a special-occasion dish, these succulent game hens can't be beat. Serve with *Vegetable Medley (page 151).*

| TOTAL CARBOHYDRATES: *2 grams* |
| PER SERVING: *1 gram* |

3 tablespoons butter
2 Cornish game hens,
   quartered
¼ cup dry white wine

juice of ½ lime
⅓ cup chicken stock
salt and pepper to taste

• Heat the butter in a heavy casserole or Dutch oven over medium-high heat until the foam subsides. Add the hens and cook for 5 minutes on each side. Add the wine, lime juice, chicken stock, salt, and pepper, and bring to a boil. Lower the heat to medium, partially cover the casserole, and cook for 15 minutes, or until the hens are cooked through. Serve immediately.

Serves 2

• Breast of Duck with •
Red Wine Sauce

Sliced duck drizzled with a rich wine sauce makes a sophisticated main course for a formal dinner. The recipe can be doubled or tripled according to the number of guests. Serve with Green Beans with Anchovy Sauce (page 145).

> TOTAL CARBOHYDRATES: *13 grams*
>
> PER SERVING: *6.5 grams*

1 whole boneless duck breast	1 tablespoon soy sauce
1 tablespoon butter	1 tablespoon Worcestershire
1 large shallot, minced	sauce
$^{1}/_{2}$ cup dry red wine	1 beef bouillon cube
1 tablespoon balsamic vinegar	$^{1}/_{4}$ cup heavy cream

• **Prick the duck all over with a fork. Heat a nonstick skillet over medium-high heat until hot. Place the duck, skin side down, in the skillet and cook for 8 to 10 minutes, or until the skin is crisp and brown. Turn the duck and cook for another 5 minutes. Remove the duck from the skillet and keep warm.**

Heat the butter in the skillet over medium heat until the foam subsides. Add the minced shallot and cook about 1 minute, until barely golden. Add the wine, vinegar, soy sauce, Worcestershire sauce, and bouillon cube. Bring to a boil, lower the heat, and simmer for 5 minutes. Add the cream and cook over medium heat, stirring occasionally, for 2 minutes, or until the sauce is heated through (do not let it boil). Cut the duck into thin slices, arrange them on 2 plates, and top with sauce. Serve immediately.

Serves 2

Pork

•

Stir-Fried Pork with Water Chestnuts

Mustard-Crusted Pork

Pork Chops with Orange and Rosemary

Pork with Chili Sauce

Pork Casserole with Tomato and Mushrooms

Pork Tenderloin Medallions with Sour Cream and Dill

Garlic Dill Meatballs

Barbecued Spareribs

Panfried Ham and Cheese "Sandwiches"

Ham Steak with Shallot Vermouth Sauce

Ham with Port Cream Sauce

· Stir-Fried Pork with · Water Chestnuts

Crunchy water chestnuts add a wonderful texture to this simple stir-fry with delicious Asian flavors.

> TOTAL CARBOHYDRATES: *14.2 grams*
>
> PER SERVING: *7.1 grams*

1 pound pork loin
2 tablespoons canola oil
1/2 cup chopped onion
1/2 tablespoon peeled and
    minced gingerroot
3 cloves garlic, minced
1/3 cup sliced water chestnuts

1/2 cup sliced mushrooms
1 tablespoon dry white wine
salt and pepper to taste
1 tablespoon toasted sesame
    oil
1 tablespoon soy sauce

• **Cut the pork into ¼-inch slices and then into thin strips.**

Heat the canola oil in a large, heavy skillet or a wok over medium-high heat until hot but not smoking. Add the pork and stir-fry for 3 to 4 minutes, or until the pork begins to brown. Add the onion, gingerroot, and garlic, and stir-fry for 1 minute. Add the water chestnuts and mushrooms, and stir-fry for 2 minutes. Add the wine, salt, pepper, sesame oil, and soy sauce, and stir-fry for 2 minutes. Serve immediately.

Serves 2

• Mustard-Crusted Pork •

Tofu flour works as a wonderful alternative for dusting and dredging your foods. It also provides the health benefits of soy without the nutritional pitfalls of overprocessed bleached white flour. Serve with Horseradish Cream (page 168).

> TOTAL CARBOHYDRATES: *5.4 grams*
>
> PER SERVING: *2.7 grams*

2 tablespoons tofu flour or soy
    flour (available at some
    natural-food stores)
1 tablespoon mustard powder
½ teaspoon white pepper
¼ cup olive oil

1 pound boneless center-cut
    pork chops, cut against
    the grain into 3 strips
    (about ⅜ inch thick)
salt to taste

• **Combine the tofu flour, mustard powder, and pepper in a bowl and mix well. Dust the pork with the flour mixture. Heat 2 tablespoons of the oil in a heavy skillet over medium heat until hot but not smoking. Add half of the pork (do not crowd the skillet) and brown for 5 minutes on each side, or until cooked through. Repeat with the remaining oil and pork. Sprinkle the pork with salt and serve immediately.**

Serves 2

• Pork Chops with Orange • and Rosemary

In this recipe, orange and mustard enliven the flavor of meaty pork chops. The sauce is so sweet and tangy that you'll never miss the traditional applesauce.

> TOTAL CARBOHYDRATES: *10.2 grams*
>
> PER SERVING: *5.1 grams*

2 center-cut pork chops (each about ¾ inch thick)
salt and pepper to taste
soy flour, tofu flour, or whey protein (all available at natural-food stores) for dusting the pork chops
2 tablespoons plus 1 teaspoon butter
3 tablespoons chopped shallots
⅓ cup dry white wine

1 teaspoon tomato paste
1 teaspoon Worcestershire sauce
1 tablespoon grated orange zest
1 teaspoon Dijon mustard
¾ teaspoon crumbled dried rosemary or 1½ teaspoons chopped fresh rosemary

• Season the pork chops with salt and pepper, and lightly dust with soy flour, shaking off any excess. Heat 2 tablespoons of the butter in a skillet over medium-high heat until the foam subsides and sauté the pork chops for 5 minutes on each side. Transfer the pork chops to a serving plate and keep warm.

Heat the remaining teaspoon of butter until the foam subsides and sauté the shallots for about 30 seconds, until softened. Add the wine, tomato paste, Worcestershire sauce, orange zest, mustard, and rosemary to the skillet. Bring to a boil, lower the heat, and simmer the sauce for 2 minutes, making sure to scrape up any brown bits from the bottom of the skillet. Pour the sauce over the pork chops and serve immediately.

Serves 2

• Pork with Chili Sauce •

Serrano chili gives this dish a wonderful southwestern flavor.
You can use beef instead of pork for a delicious variation.

> TOTAL CARBOHYDRATES: 17. 5 grams
>
> PER SERVING: 8.7 grams

1 scallion (including ¾ of the
  green part), chopped
3 cloves garlic
⅓ cup chopped green bell
  pepper
⅓ cup chopped fresh or
  canned tomatillos
  (available at specialty
  food stores) or red or
  green tomato

1 serrano chili or jalapeño
  pepper, seeded and
  chopped
½ cup beef stock
1 tablespoon fresh lime juice
2 tablespoons dry sherry
1½ pounds pork loin, cubed
1 tablespoon paprika
3 tablespoons olive oil

• Preheat the broiler.

Combine the scallion, garlic, bell pepper, tomatillos, chili, beef stock, lime juice, and sherry in a food processor and process for 1 minute, or until well blended. Transfer the mixture to a saucepan, bring to a boil, lower the heat, and simmer for 10 minutes.

Meanwhile, place the pork in a broiler pan, sprinkle with paprika and oil, and broil for 8 to 10 minutes, turning the pork to brown on all sides. Transfer the pork to a serving plate and pour the chili sauce over it. Serve immediately.

Serves 2

• Pork Casserole with Tomato • and Mushrooms

You don't have to wait for hours to savor this hearty casserole, enriched with a flavorful tomato-mushroom sauce. Serve with Sautéed Spinach with Garlic and Olive Oil (page 148).

> TOTAL CARBOHYDRATES: *21.8 grams*
>
> PER SERVING: *10.9 grams*

2 tablespoons olive oil
4 center-cut boneless pork
    chops, sliced against the
    grain into 3 pieces
1 medium onion, chopped
2 cloves garlic, minced
1 medium tomato, chopped

½ cup sliced button
    mushrooms
¼ cup chicken stock
salt and pepper to taste
¼ cup pitted Kalamata or
    Gaeta olives (optional)

• Heat the oil in a large, heavy skillet over medium-high heat until hot but not smoking. Add the pork pieces and sauté for 3 minutes on each side. Add the onion to the skillet and sauté for 3 minutes, stirring occasionally. Add the garlic, tomato, mushrooms, chicken stock, salt, and pepper, and bring to a boil. Lower the heat, cover, and simmer for 15 minutes, stirring occasionally. Uncover, stir in the olives, if using, and simmer for another 5 minutes. Serve immediately.

Serves 2

• Pork Tenderloin Medallions •
with Sour Cream and Dill

With the richness of cognac and the surprising freshness of dill, these wonderful medallions are a quick and sophisticated center-piece for any dinner.

TOTAL CARBOHYDRATES: *4.7 grams*

PER SERVING: *2.4 grams*

2 tablespoons butter
1 pound pork tenderloin,
    sliced into about six 1-
    inch-thick medallions
¼ cup chicken stock

1 tablespoon cognac
1 clove garlic, minced
¼ cup sour cream
½ teaspoon white pepper
fresh minced dill

• Heat the butter in a heavy skillet over medium-high heat until the foam subsides. Add the pork medallions and sauté about 5 minutes each side, until nicely browned. Remove the pork from the skillet and keep warm. Add the chicken stock, cognac, and garlic to the skillet, making sure to scrape up any brown bits from the bottom of the pan. Reduce the liquid for 2–3 minutes. Remove the skillet from the heat and very slowly blend in the sour cream, 1 spoonful at a time.

Return the pork to the pan, along with any juices that have accumulated on the platter. Cook the pork over medium-low heat for 2 or 3 minutes. Transfer the pork to the platter, pour the sauce over, and sprinkle with pepper and dill. Serve immediately.

Serves 2

• Garlic Dill Meatballs •

Ever since I prepared this dish for a dinner party, I've been getting requests for an encore. Serve the meatballs alone on toothpicks as an hors d'oeuvre or on a layer of Creamy Mushroom Sauce (page 170) as an entree or first course. You can double or triple the recipe as needed.

TOTAL CARBOHYDRATES:	*12.2 grams*
PER MEATBALL:	*1 gram*

1 pound ground chicken
½ pound ground pork
1 small onion, finely chopped
½ cup ground pork rinds
 (optional)
1 large egg

2 cloves garlic, minced
2 tablespoons chopped fresh
 dill
salt and pepper to taste
2 tablespoons canola oil

● Preheat the oven to 375°F.

Combine the chicken, pork, onion, pork rinds, if using, egg, garlic, dill, salt, and pepper in a bowl and mix well. Divide the mixture into twelve 2-inch meatballs.

Heat the oil in a large ovenproof skillet over medium-high heat until hot but not smoking. Brown the meatballs, turning them, about 6 minutes. Transfer the skillet to the oven and bake the meatballs, covered, for 15 minutes. Serve immediately.

Makes about 12 meatballs

• Barbecued Spareribs •

Ribs are one of my favorite indulgences on the Atkins diet. I have created a quick version that you can make even after a long day at work.

> TOTAL CARBOHYDRATES: *2 grams*
>
> PER SERVING: *1 gram*

3 pounds spareribs
2 bay leaves
2 tablespoons whole
    peppercorns
3 tablespoons butter, softened

1 tablespoon unsweetened
    ketchup (available at
    specialty-food stores)
2 teaspoons hot pepper sauce

● **Preheat the broiler.**

Place the ribs in a large pot, cover with water, and add the bay leaves and peppercorns. Bring to a boil, lower the heat, cover, and simmer for 20 minutes.

Meanwhile, combine the butter, ketchup, and hot pepper sauce in a small bowl. Drain the ribs. Pat the butter mixture on all sides of the ribs and broil the ribs for 2 to 3 minutes on each side, or until browned and crisp. Serve immediately.

Serves 2

· Panfried Ham and · Cheese "Sandwiches"

These panfried "sandwiches" are easy and fun to prepare. Serve them with Cilantro-Lime Pesto (page 161) as a condiment.

TOTAL CARBOHYDRATES:

with Breading I (Pork Rind–Sesame Breading): 3.4 grams

with Breading II (Sesame-Tofu Breading): 7.2 grams

with Breading III (Pork Rind–Tofu Breading): 3.5 grams

PER SERVING:

with Breading I: 1.7 grams

with Breading II: 3.6 grams

with Breading III: 1.8 grams

⅓ cup breading (I, II, or III; see pages 190–192)
salt and pepper to taste
1 whole skinless, boneless chicken breast, halved
2 slices Swiss cheese
2 thin slices boiled or baked ham
2 eggs, lightly beaten
2 tablespoons olive oil

- Place the flour on a plate and season it with salt and pepper. Pound the chicken until very thin, about ⅛ of an inch thick. Place 1 slice of Swiss cheese and 1 slice of ham on each chicken piece. Fold the chicken in half, creating a half-moon. Dip the chicken in the eggs and dredge in the flour, shaking off any excess.

Heat the oil in a skillet over medium-high heat until hot but not smoking. Add the chicken and cook for 4 or 5 minutes on each side, or until golden brown. Serve immediately.

Serves 2

• Ham Steak with Shallot •
Vermouth Sauce

Precooked ham steak makes a perfect quick dinner. Try to find reduced-salt ham for the best flavor.

> TOTAL CARBOHYDRATES: *11.9 grams*
>
> PER SERVING: *5.9 grams*

1 tablespoon butter	2 tablespoons dry vermouth
1 pound precooked ham steak	1 tablespoon cognac
4 shallots, chopped	1 tablespoon balsamic vinegar
3 whole cloves	

• Heat the butter in a heavy skillet over medium heat until the foam subsides. Add the ham steak, shallots, and cloves, keeping the shallots to the side of the skillet. Cook the ham steak, stirring the shallots frequently, for 3 minutes on each side. Transfer the ham to a serving plate and keep warm.

Add the vermouth, cognac, and vinegar to the skillet. Bring to a boil, making sure to scrape up any brown bits from the bottom of the skillet. Lower the heat and simmer for 1 minute. Pour the sauce over the ham steak and serve immediately.

Serves 2

• Ham with Port Cream Sauce •

You won't believe how easy it is to dress up convenient precooked ham steaks with this rich port sauce. You can use leftover ham in this dish with great results.

TOTAL CARBOHYDRATES: *14.2 grams*

PER SERVING: *7.1 grams*

1 tablespoon butter
3 tablespoons minced shallots
1/3 cup dry white wine
3 tablespoons port wine
1 pound reduced-salt cooked
    ham steak

1 teaspoon tomato paste
1/2 cup heavy cream
salt and pepper to taste

•   Heat the butter in a skillet over medium heat until the foam subsides. Add the shallots and cook until translucent, about 2 minutes. Add the white wine, port wine, and ham to the skillet. Bring to a boil, lower the heat, and simmer for 3 minutes. Remove the ham from the skillet and keep warm.

Whisk the tomato paste and cream into the skillet, bring to a gentle boil, and simmer about 4 minutes, until slightly thickened. Season with salt and pepper. Transfer the ham to a serving plate and pour the sauce over it. Serve immediately.

Serves 2

Lamb

•

Broiled Marinated Lamb Chops
Grilled Lemon and Rosemary Lamb
Rack of Lamb with Brussels Sprouts
Braised Lamb with Cumin and Lemon
Lamb with Cabbage

• Broiled Marinated Lamb Chops •

Simple and scrumptious, these lamb chops burst with the zesty flavor of the marinade, which also gives them a wonderful glaze-like crust. Serve with Red Pepper Puree (page 158).

> TOTAL CARBOHYDRATES: *2.7 grams*
>
> PER SERVING: *1.4 grams*

2 tablespoons olive oil
1 tablespoon Worcestershire
    sauce
2 tablespoons lime juice
2 tablespoons soy sauce

2 tablespoons dry white wine
3 cloves garlic, minced
salt and pepper to taste
1 pound lamb chops (each
    about ¾ inch thick)

● **Preheat the broiler.**

Whisk together the oil, Worcestershire sauce, lime juice, soy sauce, wine, garlic, salt, and pepper in a large bowl. Add the lamb chops and let them marinate, covered, in the refrigerator for 15 minutes or up to 1 hour.

Remove the lamb chops from the marinade and pat dry. Broil the lamb chops for 4 minutes on each side for medium-rare, or until desired doneness. Serve immediately.

Serves 2

• Grilled Lemon and •
Rosemary Lamb

Lamb is one of Dr. Atkins' favorite dishes, and this rendition could not be simpler. The marinade coats each piece of lamb, making it succulent and flavorful. If you do not have a grill, you can cook the lamb under the broiler.

> TOTAL CARBOHYDRATES: 7.7 grams
>
> PER SERVING: 3.8 grams

5 tablespoons fresh lemon
    juice
½ cup olive oil
1 tablespoon fresh rosemary or
    1½ teaspoons dried
    rosemary

1 clove garlic, minced
2 teaspoons grated lemon zest
1 pound boneless lamb chops,
    cut into 1-inch cubes

● Preheat the grill or broiler.

Whisk together the lemon juice, oil, rosemary, garlic, and lemon zest in a bowl. Add the lamb and toss gently, making sure each piece is well coated. Cover and put in the refrigerator for 10 to 15 minutes. Thread the lamb onto skewers and grill or broil, turning once, for 12 minutes for medium. Serve immediately.

Serves 2

Rack of Lamb with • Brussels Sprouts

Dramatic rack of lamb is a perfect entree for a special occasion. You can double or triple the recipe for an elegant dinner party.

> TOTAL CARBOHYDRATES: *15.3 grams*
>
> PER SERVING: *7.7 grams*

1 cup stemmed fresh brussels sprouts, quartered
1 tablespoon olive oil
1 tablespoon coriander seeds
1 tablespoon chopped fresh rosemary or 1½ teaspoons crumbled dried rosemary

2 tablespoons peppercorns
2 cloves garlic
1 pound rack of lamb (about 6 ribs), cut in half
1 tablespoon Dijon mustard
salt to taste

● **Preheat the oven to 425°F.**

Place the brussels sprouts in a roasting pan and sprinkle with the oil. Place the coriander, rosemary, peppercorns, and garlic in a food processor and blend for 10 seconds. Brush the lamb with the mustard, then pat it with the pepper mixture, coating the lamb, and sprinkle with salt. Arrange the lamb on top of the brussels sprouts in the roasting pan and roast for 25 minutes for rare, 30 to 35 minutes for medium. Serve immediately.

Serves 2

• Braised Lamb with Cumin • and Lemon

When lamb is braised with spices, it becomes infused with flavor. This dish is made with the neck bone of the lamb, an inexpensive but extremely tender cut. The tasty lamb requires only thirty minutes of braising, but if you have the time, you can braise it for up to an hour for added flavor. Serve it with Mint Cumin Pesto (page 162) as a condiment on the side.

> TOTAL CARBOHYDRATES: 14.8 grams
>
> PER SERVING: 7.4 grams

1 tablespoon olive oil
2 pounds neck of lamb, cut into 2-inch pieces, or 1½ pounds lamb shoulder, cut into 1-inch cubes
2 tablespoons tofu or soy flour (available at natural-food stores)
1 teaspoon ground cumin
1 teaspoon ground turmeric
2 teaspoons ground coriander
3 cloves garlic, minced
½ cup chicken stock
juice of 1 lemon
¼ cup sour cream
salt to taste

• Heat the oil in a large casserole over medium-high heat until hot but not smoking. Dust the lamb with the flour and sauté in a single layer for 3 to 4 minutes on each side, or until browned. Add the cumin, turmeric, coriander, garlic, chicken stock, and lemon juice. Cover the casserole tightly and braise over low heat for 30 minutes. Stir in the sour cream and salt during the last 5 minutes of cooking. Serve immediately.

Serves 2

• Lamb with Cabbage •

Cabbage becomes very sweet when it is simmered. In this dish the cabbage lends a wonderful flavor to the lamb.

TOTAL CARBOHYDRATES: 20.5 grams

PER SERVING: 10.3 grams

2 tablespoons olive oil
1 tablespoon butter
1 1/2 pounds lamb shoulder, cut
    into 2 or 3 pieces
1 tablespoon paprika
1/2 small head cabbage, thinly
    sliced

1/2 cup chopped onion
3 cloves garlic, minced
1/4 cup dry white wine
2 tablespoons heavy cream
salt and pepper to taste

• Heat the oil and butter in a large, heavy skillet over medium heat until the foam subsides. Add the lamb and paprika, and brown the lamb on all sides, about 8 minutes. Remove the lamb from the skillet.

Add the cabbage, onion, and garlic to the skillet and cook for 2 minutes, stirring occasionally. Place the lamb on top of the cabbage mixture, add the wine, and bring to a boil. Lower the heat, cover, and simmer for 5 minutes. Stir in the cream, salt, and pepper, and cook, uncovered, for 2 minutes. Serve immediately.

Serves 2

Veal

•

Veal Saltimbocca
Veal Scallops with Wine and Mushrooms
Veal Stuffed with Ham, Gruyère, and Bacon

• Veal Saltimbocca •

Here's a delicious Italian classic that's easy to prepare and makes a lovely presentation.

> TOTAL CARBOHYDRATES: *8.4 grams*
>
> PER SERVING: *4.2 grams*

*½ pound veal scallops,
        pounded to a ⅛-inch
        thickness*
salt and pepper to taste
*soy flour, tofu flour, or whey
        protein (all available at
        natural-food stores) for
        dusting the veal*
4 tablespoons (½ stick) butter

¼ cup grated Parmesan cheese
4 thin slices prosciutto
*1 tablespoon Worcestershire
        sauce*
⅓ cup dry white wine
*1 tablespoon chopped fresh
        sage leaves or 1½
        teaspoons crumbled dried
        sage*

• **Preheat the oven to 375°F.**

Season the veal with salt and pepper, and lightly dust with the soy flour, shaking off any excess. Heat 3 tablespoons of the butter in a large skillet over medium-high heat until the foam subsides. Sauté the veal for 1 minute on each side. Transfer the veal to a baking sheet.

Sprinkle the Parmesan evenly over the veal and top each veal scallop with a piece of prosciutto, cut to fit the size of the veal. Bake for 5 minutes. While the veal is baking, add the Worcestershire, wine, and sage to the skillet. Bring to a boil, making sure to scrape up any brown bits from the bottom of the skillet. Lower the heat and simmer for 2 minutes. Remove from the heat and whisk in the remaining tablespoon of butter. Transfer the veal to a serving plate, pour the sauce over it, and serve immediately.

Serves 2

· Veal Scallops with Wine · and Mushrooms

The tang of lemon and the earthiness of sautéed mushrooms complement these delicate veal scallops. Serve with Sautéed Zucchini with Nutmeg (page 142).

> TOTAL CARBOHYDRATES: *18 grams*
>
> PER SERVING: *9 grams*

1 tablespoon butter
1 tablespoon olive oil
1/3 cup chopped scallions
    (white part only)
2 cups sliced mushrooms
3/4 pound veal scallops,
    pounded to a 1/8-inch
    thickness

1/2 cup dry white wine
1 tablespoon cognac
4 teaspoons lemon juice
salt and pepper to taste

● Heat the butter and oil in a skillet over medium-high heat until the foam subsides. Add the scallions and mushrooms, and sauté for 4 minutes, stirring occasionally. Push the mushroom mixture to the side of the skillet, add the veal, and sauté for 1 minute on each side. Transfer the veal to a plate and keep warm.

Add the wine, cognac, lemon juice, salt, and pepper to the skillet. Bring to a boil, lower the heat, and simmer for 2 minutes. Pour the sauce over the veal and serve immediately.

Serves 2

Veal Stuffed with Ham, Gruyère, and Bacon

For a hearty dinner, this richly stuffed veal with wine sauce is one of our favorites. When accompanied by our Broccoli Puree with Garlic (page 146), it becomes the epitome of the luxurious foods we can enjoy on the low-carbohydrate diet.

> TOTAL CARBOHYDRATES: *13.8 grams*
>
> PER SERVING: *6.5 grams*

4 thinly sliced veal cutlets
(about ¼ pound each)
2 thin slices prepared ham
(boiled or baked)
2 thin slices of Gruyère cheese
2 strips bacon, halved and
cooked
4 tablespoons (½ stick) butter

1 tablespoon olive oil
1 tablespoon minced shallots
½ cup thinly sliced mushrooms
½ cup white wine
½ cup chicken stock
½ teaspoon ground white
pepper

• Pound the veal cutlets until very thin. Place 2 veal cutlets on a work surface and top each cutlet with 1 slice of ham, 1 slice of Gruyère, and 2 pieces of bacon. (Be sure the filling does not extend over the edges of the veal.) Top each cutlet with another slice of veal and secure the edges with small skewers.

Heat the butter and oil in a skillet over medium heat until hot but not smoking. Add the cutlets and cook for about 4 minutes on each side. Remove from the skillet and keep warm on a platter. Add shallots, mushrooms, wine, stock, and pepper to the skillet. Reduce the liquid over medium-high heat for 2 minutes, making sure to scrape up any brown bits in the skillet. Pour the sauce over the veal and serve immediately.

Serves 2

Beef

•

Spiced Skirt Steak

Filets Mignons with Zesty Wine Sauce

Rib-eye Steak with Red Wine Sauce

Sirloin Steak with Cognac Mustard Sauce

Steak au Poivre

Beef Burgers with Feta and Tomato

Chevapchichi (Spicy Meat Rolls)

Quick and Easy Beef Goulash

Combo Curry

Meat-izza (Crustless Pizza)

· Spiced Skirt Steak ·

Simple and flavorful, this quick-to-fix skirt steak is a great staple for the Atkins diet. Serve it with Roasted Peppers in Garlic Oil (page 150) or try tossing the sliced steak with baby greens and your favorite homemade dressing.

> TOTAL CARBOHYDRATES: 2.7 grams
>
> PER SERVING: 1.4 grams

1 teaspoon paprika
1 teaspoon cumin
1 teaspoon ground coriander

salt and pepper to taste
1 pound skirt steak

- Preheat the grill or broiler.

Combine the paprika, cumin, coriander, salt, and pepper in a small bowl. Rub the spice mixture over the entire surface of the steak and let the steak marinate, covered with plastic wrap, in the refrigerator for 20 minutes.

Grill or broil the steak for 2½ to 3 minutes on each side for medium-rare. Let stand for 5 minutes.

Cut the steak diagonally into thin slices. Serve immediately or store in the refrigerator, wrapped well, for up to 2 days.

Serves 2

· Filets Mignons with ·
Zesty Wine Sauce

Filets mignons make the perfect elegant dinner for two. In this recipe the zestiness of the red wine sauce contrasts beautifully with the tender beef. Serve Fennel Salad with Parmesan (page 50) as a starter.

> TOTAL CARBOHYDRATES: 9.3 grams
>
> PER SERVING: 4.7 grams

1 cup dry red wine
juice of 1 lime
¼ cup plus 1 tablespoon olive oil
3 cloves garlic, minced
½ teaspoon freshly ground pepper

½ cup beef stock
4 filets mignons (each about ¾ inch thick)
2 tablespoons butter
4 oil-packed anchovy fillets, mashed
2 tablespoons sour cream

- Whisk together the wine, lime juice, ¼ cup of oil, garlic, pepper, and beef stock in a large bowl. Add the filets mignons to the marinade and let stand for 10 minutes. Heat the butter and remaining tablespoon of oil in a heavy skillet over medium-high heat until hot but not smoking. Remove the filets from the marinade and pat dry. Reserve the marinade. Sauté the filets for 4 minutes on each side for medium-rare. Transfer the filets to a plate and keep warm.

Add the reserved marinade and anchovies to the skillet and boil, stirring frequently, for 5 minutes. Whisk in the sour cream and cook over low heat for 2 minutes, or until the sauce is heated through (do not let it boil). Pour the sauce over the filets and serve immediately.

Serves 2

• Rib-eye Steak with •
Red Wine Sauce

This rich, comforting dish is perfect for the colder months. If you have access to fresh herbs, add some chopped tarragon or rosemary to the sauce. Serve with Broccoli Puree with Garlic (page 146) for an elegant entree at a candlelit dinner.

> TOTAL CARBOHYDRATES: 13 grams
>
> PER SERVING: 6.5 grams

2 tablespoons olive oil
1 pound boneless rib-eye steak
    (about ½ inch thick)
1 tablespoon butter
2 large cloves garlic, minced
3 tablespoons minced shallots

½ cup red wine
¼ cup beef stock
¼ teaspoon freshly ground
    pepper
salt to taste

• Heat the oil in a large, heavy skillet over medium-high heat until hot but not smoking. Lower the heat to medium, add the steak, and cook for 6 minutes on each side for medium. Remove the steak from the skillet and keep warm.

Heat the butter in the skillet until the foam subsides. Add the garlic and shallots, and cook, stirring, for 3 minutes, or until the shallots become transparent. Add the wine, stock, pepper, and salt. Bring to a boil, making sure to scrape up any brown bits from the bottom of the skillet. Lower the heat and simmer for 3 minutes. Slice the steak into thin strips and top with the wine sauce. Serve immediately.

Serves 2

· Sirloin Steak with ·
Cognac Mustard Sauce

This elegant dish can be prepared in only fifteen minutes. It makes the perfect romantic dinner entree for two.

> TOTAL CARBOHYDRATES: 8.7 grams
>
> PER SERVING: 4.3 grams

1 1/2 pounds boneless sirloin
    steak (about 3/8 inch
    thick)
4 tablespoons (1/2 stick) butter
1/4 cup heavy cream

3 tablespoons cognac
1 tablespoon Dijon mustard
2 tablespoons Worcestershire
    sauce
salt and pepper to taste

• Cut the steak into 4 pieces. Place each piece between 2 sheets of plastic wrap and pound until thin, about 1/8 inch thick. Heat 2 tablespoons of the butter in a large, heavy skillet over medium-high heat until the foam subsides. Sauté the steak, in batches if necessary (do not crowd the skillet), for about 45 seconds on each side. Transfer the steak to a serving plate and keep warm.

Add the remaining butter, cream, cognac, mustard, Worcestershire sauce, salt, and pepper to the skillet. Bring to a boil, lower the heat, and simmer the sauce for 3 minutes, making sure to scrape up any brown bits from the bottom of the skillet. Pour the sauce over the steak and serve immediately.

Serves 2

• Steak au Poivre •

Steak au poivre is one of the great indulgences of the low-carbohydrate diet. The combination of peppercorns, cognac, and cream
is sophisticated and flavorful. We have added a touch of unsweetened ketchup, which imparts a lovely color and a hint of fruiti-
ness to this classic dish.

> TOTAL CARBOHYDRATES: 9.4 grams
>
> PER SERVING: 4.7 grams

2 tablespoons crushed
    peppercorns (see Hint)
2 boneless sirloin shell steaks
    (each about 1 inch
    thick)
2 tablespoons olive oil

½ cup heavy cream
1 tablespoon unsweetened
    ketchup (available at
    natural-food stores)
1 tablespoon cognac
salt to taste

• Spread the peppercorns on a work surface and press both
sides of the steaks into the peppercorns so that the steaks are well
coated. Heat the oil in a large, heavy skillet over medium-high
heat until hot but not smoking. Add the steaks and cook for 5
minutes on each side for medium-rare. Remove the steaks from
the skillet and keep warm.

Add the cream, ketchup, cognac, and salt to the skillet. Bring
to a boil, stirring, and making sure to scrape up any brown bits
from the bottom of the skillet. Lower the heat and simmer the
sauce for 2 minutes. Pour the sauce over the steaks and serve immediately.

Serves 2

Hint:

To crush peppercorns, place the peppercorns in a plastic bag and
flatten them with a rolling pin or the flat side of a knife.

• Beef Burgers with • Feta and Tomato

Think of these burgers as mini—meat loaves with lots of flavors. They are great on the grill and equally delicious panfried. Serve with Creamy Celery Sauce (page 167) or Cucumber-Dill Sauce (page 166).

> TOTAL CARBOHYDRATES: 9.5 grams
>
> PER SERVING: 4.8 grams

1 pound ground beef (round or chuck)

1½ teaspoons chopped fresh thyme leaves or ¾ teaspoon crumbled dried thyme

1 scallion (white part only), chopped

½ cup chopped fresh spinach

¼ cup chopped tomato

2 ounces crumbled feta cheese

salt and pepper to taste

1 teaspoon chopped fresh mint leaves (optional)

• **Combine the ground beef, thyme, scallion, spinach, tomato, feta, salt, pepper, and mint, if desired, in a large bowl and mix well. Form into 2 patties. Grill or panfry over medium-high heat for 5 minutes on each side for medium-rare, or until desired doneness. Serve immediately.**

Serves 2

• Chevapchichi (Spicy Meat Rolls) •

They're not your mother's meatballs. Flavorful and rich, these hot and spicy meat rolls pair nicely with our refreshing chilled Cucumber-Dill Sauce (page 166).

> TOTAL CARBOHYDRATES: *11.6 grams*
>
> PER SERVING: *5.8 grams*

½ pound ground veal
½ pound ground beef
½ pound ground pork
2 tablespoons club soda
½ medium onion, finely
    chopped
2 cloves garlic, minced
1 tablespoon finely chopped
    fresh flat-leaf parsley

1 teaspoon Hungarian
    paprika
½ teaspoon freshly ground
    pepper
2 tablespoons olive oil
salt to taste

•   Combine the veal, beef, pork, club soda, onion, garlic, parsley, paprika, and pepper in a large bowl and mix well. Take 1 heaping tablespoon of the mixture and shape it into a 3-inch roll. Continue making rolls in the same manner until all the mixture is used. (You will have 15 to 20 rolls.)

Heat the oil in a heavy skillet over medium heat until it is hot but not smoking. Cook the rolls in batches, turning them frequently, about 12 to 15 minutes, until nicely browned. Sprinkle the rolls with salt and serve immediately.

Serves 2—4

• Quick and Easy Beef Goulash •

When I succeeded in developing a recipe for a quick beef goulash, I was thrilled. And even though this stew takes less than thirty minutes, it still has that rich braised flavor.

TOTAL CARBOHYDRATES: *19.3 grams*

PER SERVING: *9.7 grams*

2 scallions (white part only)
3 large cloves garlic
1 large tomato
3 tablespoons olive oil
1½ pounds boneless sirloin,
    cut into ¾-inch cubes

2 teaspoons paprika
salt and pepper to taste
¼ cup heavy cream
1 cube beef bouillon

• Combine the scallions, garlic, and tomato in a food processor and puree for 1 minute, or until smooth. Heat 1 tablespoon of the oil in a saucepan over medium heat until hot but not smoking. Add the tomato mixture and cook, stirring occasionally, for 5 minutes.

Season the sirloin with the paprika, salt, and pepper. Heat the remaining 2 tablespoons of oil in a large, deep skillet over medium-high heat until hot but not smoking. Brown the meat, in batches if necessary, about 5 to 7 minutes.

Pour the tomato mixture over the meat and cook over medium-high heat, stirring occasionally, for 10 minutes. Stir in the cream and bouillon, and cook for 2 minutes, or until heated through (do not let the goulash boil). Serve immediately.

Serves 2

· Combo Curry ·

Don't throw away those leftover meats! Toss them into this quick-to-fix curry.

> TOTAL CARBOHYDRATES: *17.6 grams*
>
> PER SERVING: *8.8 grams*

1 tablespoon butter
1 tablespoon canola oil
½ cup chopped onion
2 cloves garlic, minced
1 tablespoon curry powder
½ cup water
¼ cup heavy cream
1½ teaspoons peeled and
    chopped fresh gingerroot

½ chicken bouillon cube
2 cups cubed leftover meats
    (such as a combination
    of beef and pork or
    chicken and turkey)
2 tablespoons chopped
    walnuts, lightly toasted
    (see Hint on page 163)

● **Heat the butter and oil in a large, heavy skillet over medium-high heat until the foam subsides. Add the onion, garlic, and curry powder, and sauté, stirring occasionally, for 3 to 4 minutes, or until the onion is wilted. Add the water, cream, gingerroot, and bouillon. Bring to a gentle boil and simmer for 5 minutes. Add the leftover meats and cook over medium heat, stirring occasionally, for 5 minutes, or until heated through. Sprinkle with the walnuts and serve immediately.**

Serves 2

• Meat-izza • (Crustless Pizza)

We have created a "crust" of ground beef for this Atkins pizza. Be careful when you remove the pizza from the pan because the meat may crumble—but it is still delicious.

> TOTAL CARBOHYDRATES: 15.6 grams
>
> PER SERVING: 7.6 grams

3/4 pound ground beef
3 cloves garlic, minced
2 tablespoons ground hazelnuts
1/2 cup chicken bouillon
1/2 tablespoon fennel seeds, crushed
1/4 sugarless medium-hot salsa

3/4 cup shredded mozzarella cheese
1/4 cup grated Parmesan cheese
1 tablespoon chopped fresh basil or 1 1/2 teaspoons crumbled dried basil
1 teaspoon dried oregano
salt and pepper to taste

- Preheat the oven to 400°F.

Combine the beef, garlic, hazelnuts, chicken bouillon, and fennel seeds in a large bowl and mix well. Transfer the beef mixture to a 9-inch pie pan. Spread it evenly over the bottom and halfway up the side of the pan, and bake for 12 minutes. Remove from the oven and pour off any accumulated juices. Spread the salsa over the meat and top with the mozzarella, Parmesan, basil, oregano, salt, and pepper. Return to the oven and bake for 10 minutes. Preheat the broiler and broil the pizza for 3 minutes, or until the cheese is melted and browned. Serve immediately.

Serves 2

Vegetables

•

Cauliflower with Cumin Seed

Cauliflower and Mushroom Puree

Cucumber in Cream Sauce

Sautéed Zucchini with Nutmeg

Wax Beans with Garlic-Tarragon Vinaigrette

Snow Peas with Hazelnuts

Green Beans with Anchovy Sauce

Broccoli Puree with Garlic

Broccoli Rabe with Spicy Sausage

Sautéed Spinach with Garlic and Olive Oil

Pureed Avocado with Garlic and Tarragon

Roasted Peppers in Garlic Oil

Vegetable Medley

Stir-Fried Vegetables with Mustard Seeds
and Balsamic Vinegar

Spinach and Cheddar Casserole

Chiles Rellenos

• Cauliflower with Cumin Seed •

This fragrant dish can be served either hot or at room temperature. If you are not a fan of cumin seeds, you can substitute an equal amount of fennel or caraway seeds.

TOTAL CARBOHYDRATES: *16.1 grams*

PER SERVING: *8.1 grams*

2 tablespoons cumin seeds
1/4 cup olive oil
2 cloves garlic, thinly sliced

2 cups cauliflower florets, cut
into bite-size pieces
salt and pepper to taste

• **Heat a skillet over medium heat until hot but not smoking. Add the cumin seeds and cook until the seeds begin to brown and pop, about 1 minute. Remove from the skillet and reserve. Heat the oil in the same skillet, add the garlic, and sauté for 30 seconds. Add the cauliflower and sauté, stirring occasionally, about 5 minutes, until the cauliflower begins to brown. Add the toasted cumin seeds, salt, and pepper, toss well, and serve.**

Serves 2

• Cauliflower and •
Mushroom Puree

This smooth-textured puree makes a sophisticated side dish. Serve it with a simple entree such as Pork Chops with Orange and Rosemary (page 107).

> TOTAL CARBOHYDRATES: *20.1 grams*
>
> PER SERVING: *10 grams*

1½ cups chopped cauliflower
2 tablespoons olive oil
2 tablespoons butter
1 small onion, finely chopped

1½ cups sliced mushrooms
2 tablespoons crème fraîche or
    heavy cream
salt and pepper to taste

• **Bring 2 quarts of salted water to a boil in a large saucepan. Add the cauliflower and cook for 6 minutes. Drain and set aside.**

    Meanwhile, heat the oil and butter in a large skillet over medium-high heat until the foam subsides. Add the onion to the skillet and sauté for 5 minutes. Add the mushrooms and sauté, stirring occasionally, for 5 minutes.

    Transfer the cauliflower and the mushroom mixture to a food processor. Add the crème fraîche, salt, and pepper, and puree for 1 minute, or until smooth. Cook the puree in a saucepan over low heat, stirring occasionally, for 3 minutes, or until it is heated through. Serve immediately.

Serves 2

• Cucumber in Cream Sauce •

After first tasting this delightful cucumber dish at a dinner party in Denver, I created my own version. Serve with Pepper-Crusted Swordfish (page 86) or grilled salmon.

TOTAL CARBOHYDRATES: *18.4 grams*

PER SERVING: *8.7 grams*

1 tablespoon canola oil
1 tablespoon butter
1 medium leek (white part only), halved lengthwise, washed well, and thinly sliced
1 medium cucumber, peeled, seeded, and thinly sliced
2 tablespoons dry vermouth or dry sherry

1 tablespoon grated lemon zest
juice of ½ lemon
1 chicken bouillon cube
1 large basil leaf, chopped, or 1 teaspoon crumbled dried basil
salt and pepper to taste
½ cup heavy cream

• Heat the oil and butter in a skillet over medium heat until the foam subsides. Add the leek and cook, stirring occasionally, for 3 to 4 minutes, or until softened. Add the cucumber and cook for 5 minutes, stirring occasionally. Add the vermouth, lemon zest, lemon juice, bouillon, basil, salt, and pepper. Partially cover the skillet and cook for 10 minutes, stirring occasionally. Add the cream and cook for 1 minute, or until heated through. Serve immediately.

Serves 2

• Sautéed Zucchini with Nutmeg •

The delicacy of this speedy sauté makes it a perfect partner for
Mustard-Crusted Pork (page 106).

TOTAL CARBOHYDRATES:	7.7 grams
PER SERVING:	3.9 grams

2 tablespoons butter
2 medium zucchini, cut into
⅜-inch-thick slices

salt and pepper to taste
nutmeg to taste

• Heat the butter in a skillet over medium-high heat until the
foam subsides. Add the zucchini, and sauté for 10 minutes, stirring frequently. Sprinkle with salt, pepper, and nutmeg. Serve immediately.

Serves 2

· Wax Beans with ·
Garlic-Tarragon Vinaigrette

Wax beans are wonderfully flavorful when they are tossed with this simple garlic-tarragon vinaigrette. Serve as a side dish with beef or lamb.

> TOTAL CARBOHYDRATES: *16.4 grams*
>
> PER SERVING: *8.2 grams*

2 cups wax beans, trimmed
5 tablespoons olive oil
1/3 cup finely chopped onion
1 garlic clove, minced
2 tablespoons white wine
    vinegar

1 tablespoon chopped fresh
    tarragon leaves or 1 1/2
    teaspoons crumbled dried
    tarragon
salt and pepper to taste

● **Bring 2 quarts of salted water to a boil in a large saucepan. Add the wax beans and cook for 5 to 6 minutes, or until tender. Drain the wax beans and refresh them under cold water to stop the cooking. Whisk together the olive oil, onion, garlic, vinegar, tarragon, salt, and pepper.**

    Transfer the wax beans to a serving bowl. Pour the vinaigrette over them and toss well. Let the beans stand for 10 minutes. Serve immediately or store in an airtight container in the refrigerator for up to 1 day.

Serves 2

• Snow Peas with Hazelnuts •

Flavorful roasted nuts make a wonderful addition to sautéed vegetables. Hazelnuts, which are sometimes called filberts, are among our favorites.

TOTAL CARBOHYDRATES: 20.2 grams

PER SERVING: 10.1 grams

½ cup diced slab bacon
2 tablespoons butter
½ pound snow peas, washed

2 tablespoons hazelnuts,
   skinned
salt and pepper to taste

• Heat a large, heavy skillet over medium-high heat until hot. Sauté the bacon, stirring occasionally, about 2 minutes, until browned. Remove the bacon from the skillet and pour out the bacon fat. In the same skillet heat the butter over low heat until the foam subsides. Add the snow peas and cook until crisp-tender, about 1 minute.

Heat a small skillet over medium heat until hot. Add the hazelnuts and roast, shaking the skillet occasionally, for 4 to 5 minutes, until golden and aromatic. Add the bacon, snow peas, salt, and pepper, and sauté over medium-high heat for 2 minutes. Serve immediately.

Serves 2 or 3

Variation: Substitute roasted walnuts for the hazelnuts and add 1 tablespoon of minced fresh gingerroot and 1 tablespoon of soy sauce to the snow peas when adding the bacon.

• Green Beans with Anchovy Sauce •

Green beans are a great vehicle for this salty anchovy sauce. Serve as a side dish with Grilled Lemon and Rosemary Lamb (page 118).

TOTAL CARBOHYDRATES: *20 grams*

PER SERVING: *10 grams*

1 pound green beans, trimmed
   and washed
3 oil-packed anchovy fillets or
   1 tablespoon homemade
   Anchovy Paste (recipe on
   page 159) or prepared
   anchovy paste

2 tablespoons butter
$\frac{1}{2}$ cup chicken stock
1 tablespoon chopped basil for
   garnish

• Bring 2 quarts of salted water to a boil in a large saucepan. Add the green beans and cook for 5 minutes. While the beans are cooking, combine the anchovy fillets or anchovy paste, butter, and stock in a small saucepan and bring to a slow boil.

Drain the green beans and transfer them to a bowl. Pour the anchovy sauce over the beans, toss well, and garnish with the basil. Serve immediately.

Serves 2

• Broccoli Puree with Garlic •

This puree is a wonderful side dish. Sometimes we like to serve it as a bed for our Veal Stuffed with Ham, Gruyère, and Bacon (page 125). We like to mix crème fraîche into the puree for a richer side dish that can accompany simpler entrees, such as roast lamb.

> TOTAL CARBOHYDRATES: *14 grams*
>
> PER SERVING: *7 grams*

3 stalks broccoli, stems
    discarded and heads
    washed well and
    separated into florets

2 tablespoons olive oil
2 cloves garlic
salt to taste
½ teaspoon white pepper

• Bring 1 quart of salted water to a boil in a saucepan. Add the broccoli florets and cook over medium heat, covered, for 12 to 15 minutes, until tender. Drain. Combine the broccoli with the oil, garlic, salt, and pepper in a food processor and puree for about 1 minute, until smooth. Serve immediately.

Serves 2

• Broccoli Rabe with Spicy Sausage •

The slightly bitter taste of broccoli rabe is a perfect foil for spicy Italian sausage. The addition of balsamic vinegar adds a piquant tang. This dish makes a wonderful accompaniment to Broiled Marinated Lamb Chops (page 117) and can also serve as a light lunch on its own. The water that clings to the broccoli rabe after it is washed should produce the right amount of liquid for cooking.

> TOTAL CARBOHYDRATES: *21.7 grams*
>
> PER SERVING: *10.9 grams*

2 tablespoons olive oil
1 pound hot Italian sausage, casings removed
2 cloves garlic, minced
1 pound broccoli rabe, washed
1 tablespoon balsamic vinegar
1 teaspoon freshly ground black pepper
1/2 teaspoon dried hot red pepper flakes
salt to taste

• **Heat the oil in a large skillet over medium-high heat until hot but not smoking. Add the sausage and cook for 6 minutes, breaking up the lumps. Add the garlic and cook for another minute.**

Turn the heat to low and add the broccoli rabe and vinegar. (If the broccoli rabe is too dry, add 1 teaspoon of water to the skillet.) Cover and cook, stirring occasionally, for 7 minutes, or until the broccoli rabe is tender. Stir in the pepper, hot pepper flakes, and salt. Serve immediately.

Serves 2

• Sautéed Spinach with Garlic • and Olive Oil

To this classic spinach dish we have added extra garlic and the earthy hint of nutmeg. This is the perfect accompaniment for Pork Tenderloin Medallions with Sour Cream and Dill (page 110).

> TOTAL CARBOHYDRATES: 20.4 grams
>
> PER SERVING: 10.2 grams

3 tablespoons olive oil
4 large cloves garlic, sliced
1 package frozen leaf spinach, defrosted and drained
½ cube of chicken bouillon, crumbled

¼ teaspoon freshly grated nutmeg
salt and pepper to taste

• Heat the olive oil in a saucepan over moderate heat until hot but not smoking. Add the garlic and cook about 1 minute, until it begins to turn golden. Add the spinach and sprinkle with the crumbled chicken bouillon cube. Place a lid on the saucepan, leaving it slightly ajar. Cook the spinach, stirring from time to time, until the moisture has evaporated, about 2–3 minutes. Turn off the heat and mix in the nutmeg, salt, and pepper. Serve immediately.

Serves 2

• Pureed Avocado with Garlic • and Tarragon

This puree has a vibrant green color and creamy texture. It is a perfect accompaniment to shrimp cocktail or cold salmon. Sometimes we like to use it in addition to mayonnaise for seafood and tuna salads. Remember this recipe when you have an avocado that has become too soft for other dishes.

> TOTAL CARBOHYDRATES:
>
> 18.3 grams per cup

1 ripe avocado (preferably
    Haas)
1 small clove garlic, minced
1 tablespoon fresh lemon juice
    plus ½ teaspoon for
    sprinkling over the puree

1 tablespoon olive oil
¼ cup fresh tarragon leaves
salt and pepper to taste
2 tablespoons heavy cream

• Halve the avocado, remove the pit, and scoop the flesh into a food processor. Add the garlic, 1 tablespoon of lemon juice, oil, tarragon, salt, and pepper. Puree the mixture for 30 seconds, or until smooth. With the motor running, add the cream and puree for another 15 seconds. Sprinkle the remaining lemon juice over the puree to prevent discoloration. Serve immediately or store in an airtight container in the refrigerator for up to 2 days.

Makes about 1 cup

• Roasted Peppers in Garlic Oil •

Roasting peppers is really extremely simple. Once the skin is charred, it pulls off easily, leaving the wonderfully sweet flesh. We sometimes chop roasted peppers and add them to chicken salad. Or we bathe the roasted peppers in garlic and oil, as in this recipe, and serve them as an accompaniment to grilled fish.

> TOTAL CARBOHYDRATES: *11.6 grams*
>
> PER SERVING: *5.8 grams*

¾ cup olive oil
2 cloves garlic, minced

1 red bell pepper
1 green bell pepper

• **Combine the oil and garlic in a bowl.**

To roast on a gas burner: Turn the flame to medium-high. Place the peppers directly on the flame and roast them, turning with tongs, for about 10 minutes, or until the skin is completely charred. (Alternately, you can roast the peppers in a preheated 450°F. oven, turning them frequently with tongs, for about 20 minutes, or until the skin is completely charred.) Remove from the heat, place in a paper bag, and seal the bag by folding over the top. Allow the peppers to "sweat" for 2 minutes.

Remove the peppers from the bag. Under running water pull the skin off the peppers. Remove the seeds and ribs, and add the roasted peppers to the garlic oil. Serve immediately.

Serves 2

• Vegetable Medley •

The individual flavors of the vegetables remain distinct in this colorful medley. Serve with Garlic Dill Meatballs (page 111).

> TOTAL CARBOHYDRATES: *12 grams*
>
> PER SERVING: *6 grams*

2 tablespoons olive oil
1 small onion, finely chopped
½ yellow bell pepper, diced
1 cup diced zucchini
½ cup peeled, seeded, and
    diced cucumber

¼ cup chicken stock
2 cloves garlic, minced
½ teaspoon cumin
¼ teaspoon dried oregano
salt and pepper to taste

• **Heat the oil in a large skillet over medium-high heat until hot but not smoking. Add the onion, bell pepper, zucchini, and cucumber, and sauté for 5 minutes, stirring occasionally. Add the chicken stock, garlic, cumin, oregano, salt, and pepper. Bring to a boil, lower the heat, and simmer for 10 minutes, until the vegetables are tender. Serve immediately.**

Serves 2

· Stir-Fried Vegetables with · Mustard Seeds and Balsamic Vinegar

This is a delicious and easy way to prepare a variety of vegetables you may have left over in your crisper. These are our favorite ingredients, but feel free to experiment. Other vegetables that work well in this stir-fry are snow peas, cauliflower, brussels sprouts, and mushrooms.

TOTAL CARBOHYDRATES: 16.6 grams

PER SERVING: 8.3 grams

2 tablespoons olive oil
1 cup broccoli florets
1 cup string beans, with the beans halved
1 tablespoon mustard seeds

2 large cloves garlic, diced
½ teaspoon ground pepper
1 tablespoon balsamic vinegar
salt to taste

● Heat a large, heavy skillet or wok over medium-high heat about 1 minute, until hot, and add the oil. Add the broccoli, string beans, mustard seeds, garlic, pepper, vinegar, and salt. Stir-fry the vegetables, stirring frequently, for about 10 minutes, or until tender. Serve hot or at room temperature.

Serves 2

• Spinach and Cheddar Casserole •

This rich, bubbly casserole pairs beautifully with simple grilled meat or chicken.

> **TOTAL CARBOHYDRATES: 20.7 grams**
>
> **PER SERVING: 10.4 grams**

1 tablespoon olive oil
2 garlic cloves, minced
2 pounds spinach, stemmed,
    washed, and spun dry

2 tablespoons pine nuts
1/2 cup grated cheddar cheese

● **Preheat the broiler.**

Heat the oil in a large skillet over medium heat until hot but not smoking. Add the garlic and cook for 1 minute, stirring occasionally. Add the spinach, cover, and cook for 5 minutes.

Transfer the spinach mixture to a small flameproof casserole and sprinkle with the pine nuts and cheddar. Broil the casserole until the cheese is melted and lightly browned, about 2 minutes. Serve immediately.

Serves 2

• Chiles Rellenos •

We like to add the jalapeño to these mild stuffed chilies for some kick, but they are just as delicious without it.

> **TOTAL CARBOHYDRATES:**
>
> with Breading I (Pork Rind–Sesame Breading): 19 grams
>
> with Breading II (Sesame-Tofu Breading): 22.8 grams
>
> with Breading III (Pork Rind–Tofu Breading): 19.1 grams
>
> **PER SERVING:**
>
> with Breading I: 9.5 grams
>
> with Breading II: 11.4 grams
>
> with Breading III: 9.6 grams

4 mild California chilies
　　(preferably Anaheim) or
　　Italian frying peppers
²/₃ cup grated Monterey Jack
　　cheese
²/₃ cup grated cheddar cheese
1 tablespoon seeded and
　　chopped jalapeño pepper
　　(optional)

1 large egg, lightly beaten
¼ cup breading (I, II, or III;
　　pages 190–192)
2 tablespoons canola oil

● **Blanch the chilies in boiling salted water for 5 minutes. Cool under running water. Cut open 1 side of the chilies, core, and remove the seeds, keeping the chili whole. Combine the Monterey Jack, cheddar, and jalapeño, if using, in a bowl. Stuff the chilies with the cheese mixture.**

Gently dip the chilies into the egg and dredge them in the breading, shaking off any excess. Heat the oil in a heavy skillet over medium-high heat until hot but not smoking. Add the chilies and cook until brown on all sides, about 3 minutes per side. Serve immediately.

Serves 2

Sauces

•

Sorrel Sauce

Red Pepper Puree

Anchovy Paste

Basil Pesto

Cilantro-Lime Pesto

Mint-Cumin Pesto

Walnut and Blue Cheese Butter

Zesty Cilantro Butter

Peanut Dipping Sauce

Cucumber-Dill Sauce

Creamy Celery Sauce

Horseradish Cream

Caper Tartar Sauce

Creamy Mushroom Sauce

Quick and Easy Hollandaise

• Sorrel Sauce •

Sorrel—a slightly sour herb that has grown wild for centuries throughout North America, Europe, and Asia—is available in limited supply all year. It is worth seeking out, especially in the spring, when it is at its youngest and mildest. If you can't find sorrel, you can substitute arugula. Serve this elegant sauce with fish or chicken.

> TOTAL CARBOHYDRATES:
>
> 13.6 grams per cup (if using sorrel)
> 7.9 grams per cup (if using arugula)

1 cup chicken stock	2 tablespoons chopped fresh
3 cups trimmed sorrel, washed	dill
well	salt and pepper to taste
¼ cup heavy cream	

• **Bring the chicken stock to a boil in a heavy saucepan over medium-high heat. Turn the heat to low, add the sorrel, and simmer for 15 minutes, or until the sorrel is very wilted. Add the cream, dill, salt, and pepper, and cook for 1 minute, or until the sauce is heated through (do not let it boil). Serve immediately.**

Makes about 1 cup

• Red Pepper Puree •

This puree is always a big hit, and it is shamefully simple. Serve it with grilled or blackened tuna steaks. You can also thin the puree with some chicken stock to make a sprightly soup, which can be served warm or chilled.

> **TOTAL CARBOHYDRATES:**
>
> *17.9 per 1½ cups*

1½ tablespoons olive oil
1 red bell pepper, chopped
1 roasted red bell pepper
  (procedure on page
  150), chopped, or ½ cup
  chopped bottled roasted
  red pepper
2 cloves garlic, chopped

½ cup chopped onion
2 tablespoons red wine
1½ teaspoons fresh lemon
  juice
1 tablespoon fresh tarragon
  leaves (optional)
salt and pepper to taste

• Heat the oil in a heavy skillet over medium heat until hot but not smoking. Add the peppers, garlic, onion, and wine. Cover and cook for 6 minutes, stirring occasionally. (If the liquid begins to evaporate, add 1 to 2 tablespoons of water.) Remove from the heat and transfer to a food processor. Add the lemon juice, tarragon, salt, and pepper, and puree for 30 seconds, or until smooth. Taste and adjust the seasoning. Serve immediately or store in an airtight container in the refrigerator for up to 3 days.

Makes about 1½ cups

• Anchovy Paste •

Even though anchovy paste is available ready-made, we prefer to make it ourselves so we can control the saltiness. We keep it on hand for Caesar Dressing (page 178) or Green Beans with Anchovy Sauce (page 145).

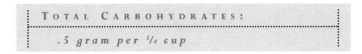

TOTAL CARBOHYDRATES:

.5 gram per ¼ cup

one 2-ounce can oil-packed
   anchovies
1 tablespoon olive oil

1½ teaspoons grated lemon
   zest

• Gently rinse the anchovies in water, pat dry, and place in a food processor. Add the oil and lemon zest, and puree for 30 seconds, or until smooth. Scrape down the side and puree for another 5 seconds. (If the puree is too chunky, add a bit more oil and puree again.) Use immediately or store in an airtight container in the refrigerator for up to 1 week.

Makes ¼ cup

• Basil Pesto •

This classic pesto is traditionally served on pasta—but not here!
Toss it with shredded cooked chicken for a lively chicken salad or
serve it as a condiment with grilled pork chops.

> TOTAL CARBOHYDRATES:
>
> 9.8 grams per ¾ cup

2 cloves garlic
1½ cups fresh basil leaves,
    washed and spun dry
3 tablespoons pine nuts

3 tablespoons grated Parmesan
    cheese
⅓ cup olive oil
salt and pepper to taste

• Place the garlic, basil leaves, pine nuts, and Parmesan in a food
processor and blend for a few seconds. Scrape down the side.
With the motor running, add the oil in a steady stream and puree
until smooth, about 1 minute. Transfer the pesto to a bowl and stir
in the salt and pepper. Serve immediately or store, covered, in the
refrigerator for up to 2 days.

Makes about ¾ cup

• Cilantro-Lime Pesto •

This pesto is divine when served with Chicken Cutlets (page 91) or grilled fish.

> TOTAL CARBOHYDRATES:
>
> 6 grams per cup

1 cup loosely packed fresh
cilantro leaves
1 clove garlic
½ tablespoon lime juice

⅓ cup coarsely chopped
walnuts
salt and pepper to taste
⅓ cup olive oil

• In a food processor, combine the cilantro, garlic, lime juice, walnuts, salt, and pepper. Process for 30 seconds and scrape down the side. With the motor running, add the oil in a slow stream and process for another 15 seconds, or until the pesto is smooth. Serve immediately or store in an airtight container in the refrigerator for up to 3 days or in the freezer for up to 2 weeks.

Makes about 1 cup

Hint:

For convenient future use, you can freeze the pesto in an ice-cube tray covered with plastic wrap.

• Mint-Cumin Pesto •

Lively mint and aromatic cumin—an unusual team—pair up
nicely in this flavorful pesto. Serve it as a condiment with lamb.

> TOTAL CARBOHYDRATES:
>
> 12.5 grams per cup

1 cup loosely packed mint
    leaves
1 clove garlic
1 1/2 teaspoons fresh lime juice
1/3 cup coarsely chopped
    walnuts, lightly toasted
    (see Hint on page 163)

1 teaspoon ground cumin
salt and pepper to taste
1/3 cup olive oil

• **In a food processor, combine the mint, garlic, lime juice, walnuts, cumin, salt, and pepper. Process for 30 seconds and scrape
down the side. With the motor running, add the oil in a slow
stream and process for another 15 seconds, or until smooth. Serve
immediately or store in an airtight container in the refrigerator
for up to 3 days or in the freezer for up to 2 weeks.**

Makes about 1 cup

• Walnut and Blue Cheese Butter •

This rich butter can turn a simple cut of beef into an elegant and sophisticated dish. We also like to combine it with cauliflower florets and bake the mixture for a creative alternative to the traditional "au gratin."

TOTAL CARBOHYDRATES: *2.7 grams*

PER SERVING: *1.3 grams*

2 ounces blue cheese, crumbled
1½ tablespoons butter,
   softened
1 teaspoon finely chopped
   fresh flat-leaf parsley
1 teaspoon finely chopped
   fresh rosemary or thyme
1 tablespoon chopped walnuts,
   toasted (see Hint)

● **Combine the blue cheese, butter, parsley, rosemary, and walnuts in a glass or ceramic bowl and mix well. Serve the butter immediately or store it, covered, in the refrigerator for up to 3 days.**

Makes about ½ cup

Hint: To toast nuts

Heat a heavy skillet over medium heat until hot. Add the nuts and cook, stirring constantly, about 3 minutes, until very aromatic and beginning to turn brown. (Be careful that the nuts do not burn.) Remove from the heat. The toasted nuts can be served immediately, dusted lightly with salt, or stored in an airtight container for up to 1 week.

• Zesty Cilantro Butter •

You can serve this wonderful butter on string beans or use it to sauté broccoli. Try it instead of plain butter on the Sesame Sour Cream Muffins (pages 186). Or liven up broiled chicken by topping it with a tablespoon or two of the butter just before the chicken has finished cooking.

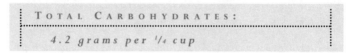

TOTAL CARBOHYDRATES:

4.2 grams per ¼ cup

3 tablespoons butter, softened

1½ tablespoons chopped fresh cilantro

1½ teaspoons grated lemon or lime zest

1 teaspoon fresh lemon or lime juice

• **Combine the butter, cilantro, zest, and lemon juice in a bowl and mix well. Serve immediately or store in an airtight container in the refrigerator for up to 1 week.**

Makes about ¼ cup

• Peanut Dipping Sauce •

This peanut dipping sauce is so tasty and easy to make. Serve it with Coconut Chicken Satés with Cilantro (page 93). You can also add a couple of tablespoons of dipping sauce to stir-fried vegetables for a distinctive Thai flavor.

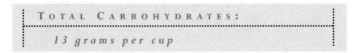

TOTAL CARBOHYDRATES:

13 grams per cup

3 tablespoons peanut butter
1 tablespoon unsweetened
   coconut milk (optional)
1 tablespoon toasted sesame
   oil

½ cup water
1 tablespoon soy sauce
juice of ½ lime
1 small clove garlic
½ cup chopped fresh cilantro

• **Combine the peanut butter, coconut milk, if using, sesame oil, water, soy sauce, lime juice, garlic, and cilantro in a food processor and puree until smooth, about 1 minute. (If the sauce is too thick, add a bit more water.) Serve immediately or store, covered, in the refrigerator for up to 4 days.**

Makes about 1 cup

• Cucumber-Dill Sauce •

We serve this wonderfully versatile sauce with our Grilled Lemon and Rosemary Lamb (page 118) or on top of a burger. You can also whisk it with some olive oil for a quick salad dressing.

> TOTAL CARBOHYDRATES:
>
> 6.2 grams per ¼ cup

¼ cup diced cucumber
½ cup sour cream
1 teaspoon fresh lemon juice
1 tablespoon chopped fresh
    dill
1 teaspoon chopped fresh mint
1 small clove garlic, minced
salt and pepper to taste

• Combine the cucumber, sour cream, lemon juice, dill, mint, garlic, salt, and pepper in a glass or ceramic bowl and mix well. Serve immediately or store in an airtight container in the refrigerator for up to 2 days.

Makes about ¾ cup

• Creamy Celery Sauce •

Serve this cool, refreshing sauce with Sautéed Sole (page 79) or Beef Burgers with Feta and Tomato (page 132). It also works well as a dip for crudités.

> TOTAL CARBOHYDRATES:
>
> 6.9 grams per ¾ cup

½ cup sour cream
¼ cup finely chopped celery
1 teaspoon ground celery seed

1½ teaspoons fresh lemon juice
salt and pepper to taste

• Whisk together the sour cream, celery, celery seed, lemon juice, salt, and pepper in a bowl until the sauce is smooth. Serve immediately or store in an airtight container in the refrigerator for up to 4 days.

Makes about ¾ cup

• Horseradish Cream •

This versatile British sauce is served traditionally over thinly sliced steak. It also makes an ideal accompaniment for cold Oven-Poached Salmon with Dill and Wine (page 82) or smoked fish.

> TOTAL CARBOHYDRATES:
>
> 4.7 grams per ¾ cup

⅓ cup heavy cream
1 teaspoon Dijon mustard
1½ tablespoons drained
    horseradish

1 tablespoon sour cream
salt and pepper to taste

• **Blend the cream and mustard in a food processor or in a bowl with an electric mixer until the mixture forms soft peaks, about 1 minute. Whisk together the horseradish, sour cream, salt, and pepper until smooth. Fold the mustard cream mixture into the horseradish mixture. Serve immediately or store in an airtight container in the refrigerator for up to 5 days.**

Makes about ¾ cup

• Caper Tartar Sauce •

Tangy capers give a wonderful flavor and texture to this home-made tartar sauce. We like ours with a dash of hot sauce, but you can adjust the "heat" according to your taste.

> TOTAL CARBOHYDRATES:
>
> 3.1 grams per ¾ cup

½ cup mayonnaise
1 tablespoon small capers or
    chopped large capers
1 teaspoon Dijon mustard
1 teaspoon drained
    horseradish

1½ teaspoons fresh lemon
    juice
1 teaspoon grated onion
salt and pepper to taste
dash of hot pepper sauce
    (optional)

• In a bowl, whisk together the mayonnaise, capers, mustard, horseradish, lemon juice, onion, salt, pepper, and hot pepper sauce, if using, until smooth. Serve immediately or store in an air-tight container in the refrigerator for up to 5 days.

Makes about ¾ cup

• Creamy Mushroom Sauce •

This versatile mushroom sauce makes a great flavor enhancer for simple grilled steaks and chops as well as for Garlic Dill Meatballs (page 111).

TOTAL CARBOHYDRATES:

8.2 grams per cup

1 tablespoon butter
½ pound button mushrooms,
    finely chopped
½ cup chicken stock

2 tablespoons heavy cream
1 tablespoon sour cream
salt and pepper to taste
nutmeg to taste

• Heat the butter in a skillet over medium heat until the foam subsides. Add the mushrooms and cook for 5 minutes, stirring frequently. Add the chicken stock and heavy cream, and cook for 2 minutes. Remove from the heat and stir in the sour cream, salt, pepper, and nutmeg. Serve immediately or store, covered, in the refrigerator for up to 1 day.

Makes about 1 cup

• Quick and Easy Hollandaise •

This blender version of the classic sauce is easy and delicious. Serve it with *Eggs Benedict with Spinach (page 71)* or steamed asparagus.

> TOTAL CARBOHYDRATES:
>
> *1.3 grams per ¹/₂ cup*

¹/₃ cup butter	salt to taste
2 egg yolks	cayenne pepper to taste
1 tablespoon fresh lemon juice	nutmeg to taste (optional)

• **Heat the butter in a saucepan over low heat until gently bubbling. Meanwhile, place the egg yolks in a blender or food processor and blend for a few seconds. With the motor running, add the lemon juice, salt, cayenne, and nutmeg, if using. Slowly add the melted butter in a thin stream and blend for 10 seconds, or until thickened and smooth.**

Makes about ¹/₂ cup

Dressings

•

Quick and Easy Salad Dressing
Shallot Orange Vinaigrette
Mustard Walnut Vinaigrette
Caesar Dressing
Smoked Salmon Dressing

• Quick and Easy Salad Dressing •

Bottled salad dressings often contain sugar or corn syrup, which boost the carbohydrate grams. You can make your own delicious dressing with some basic ingredients that you probably have in your pantry.

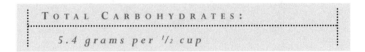

TOTAL CARBOHYDRATES:

5.4 grams per ½ cup

2 oil-packed anchovy fillets
3 tablespoons olive oil
1½ tablespoons good-quality
    vinegar (such as wine,
    balsamic, or sherry)

1 tablespoon Dijon mustard
salt and pepper to taste

● **Mash the anchovy fillets with a fork. Place in a small jar that has a tight-fitting lid. Add the oil, vinegar, mustard, salt, and pepper. Cover with the lid and shake vigorously until well blended, about 15 to 30 seconds. Serve immediately or store in the refrigerator, covered, for up to 4 days. Shake the dressing before serving.**

Makes about ½ cup

• Shallot Orange Vinaigrette •

Homemade salad dressings taste so much better than the bottled versions. This tangy, slightly sweet vinaigrette can also be used as a marinade for beef, pork, or lamb.

TOTAL CARBOHYDRATES:
13.1 grams per 1 cup

2 tablespoons balsamic
  vinegar
2 tablespoons red wine vinegar
2 teaspoons Worcestershire
  sauce
2 teaspoons Dijon mustard

1 tablespoon lime juice
1 tablespoon minced shallots
1 teaspoon grated orange zest
1 teaspoon fresh orange juice
salt and pepper to taste
¾ cup olive oil

• **In a food processor, combine the balsamic vinegar, red wine vinegar, Worcestershire sauce, mustard, lime juice, shallots, zest, orange juice, salt, and pepper, and blend for 30 seconds. With the motor running, add the oil in a slow stream and blend for another 20 seconds, or until the vinaigrette is smooth. Use immediately or store in an airtight container in the refrigerator for up to 1 week.**

Makes about 1 cup

• Mustard Walnut Vinaigrette •

A generous measure of mustard gives this vinaigrette a pungent flavor. It is a tasty alternative to mayonnaise-based dressings.

> **TOTAL CARBOHYDRATES:**
>
> 4.5 grams per ¾ cup

1½ tablespoons Dijon mustard
3 tablespoons red wine vinegar
1 small clove garlic
½ teaspoon salt
½ teaspoon freshly ground
  pepper
½ cup olive oil
1 tablespoon walnut oil

• In a food processor or blender, combine the mustard, vinegar, garlic, salt, and pepper, and blend for 30 seconds. With the motor running, add the oils in a slow stream and blend for another 10 seconds, or until the vinaigrette is smooth. Use immediately or store in an airtight container in the refrigerator for up to 1 week.

Makes about ¾ cup

• Caesar Dressing •

Because raw eggs have fallen out of favor due to the risks associated with salmonella, we have created a version of this classic dressing with a hard-boiled egg. The dressing will separate because the hard-cooked egg cannot "hold" the oil. If you prepare the dressing ahead of time, be sure to reblend it before serving.

> TOTAL CARBOHYDRATES:
>
> 4.9 grams per ¾ cup

1 hard-boiled egg, peeled
2 small cloves garlic
1½ tablespoons Anchovy Paste (page 159)
1 teaspoon fresh lemon juice
1 tablespoon Worcestershire sauce

½ teaspoon Dijon mustard
2 tablespoons olive oil
2 tablespoons grated Parmesan cheese

• Place the egg, garlic, anchovy paste, lemon juice, Worcestershire sauce, and mustard in a food processor and puree for 30 seconds, or until smooth. With the motor running, add the oil in a slow stream and then the Parmesan and puree for another 30 seconds, or until smooth. Use immediately or store in an airtight container in the refrigerator for up to 3 days. Reblend the dressing before serving.

Makes about ¾ cup

• Smoked Salmon Dressing •

This unusual dressing is great on mixed field greens. It is also delicious when served as an accompaniment to steamed asparagus or as a dip for crudités.

> **TOTAL CARBOHYDRATES:**
>
> *8.5 grams per cup*

¼ cup sour cream
½ cup mayonnaise
1½ ounces smoked salmon,
    thinly sliced
2 teaspoons white wine
    vinegar

3 teaspoons fresh lemon juice
2 tablespoons scallions (white
    part only), chopped

• **Combine the sour cream, mayonnaise, salmon, vinegar, lemon juice, and scallions in a food processor and puree for 1 minute, or until smooth. Serve immediately or store in an airtight container in the refrigerator for up to 2 days.**

Makes about 1 cup

Breads

•

Quick and Easy Bread
Cheddar Cheese Bread
Bacon Pepper Bread
Sesame Sour Cream Muffins
Savory Cheese Bites
Yorkshire Pudding
Butter Rum Muffins
Breading I
Breading II
Breading III

• Quick and Easy Bread •

Here's a moist, flavorful bread that you can make in thirty minutes.

> TOTAL AVAILABLE CARBOHYDRATES:
>
> 16.8 grams per loaf

butter for greasing the loaf pan	2 large eggs
1 cup Atkins Bake Mix*	½ cup heavy cream
	¼ cup seltzer

• **Preheat the oven to 375°F. Generously butter a loaf pan, 8½ by 4½ by 2½ inches.**

Beat together the bake mix, eggs, cream, and seltzer in a large bowl with an electric mixer. Pour the batter into the prepared pan and bake for 25 minutes. Let cool for 5 minutes. Serve immediately or store, wrapped well, in the refrigerator for up to 5 days.

Makes 1 loaf

* Available through mail order by calling 1-888-DR ATKINS.

• Cheddar Cheese Bread •

Infused with mellow cheddar, this bread is rich and satisfying.

TOTAL CARBOHYDRATES:
18 grams per loaf

butter for greasing the loaf
    pan
⅓ cup soy flour (available at
    natural-food stores)
⅓ cup whey protein (available
    at natural-food stores)

2 large eggs
½ teaspoon baking powder
2 tablespoons sour cream
2 tablespoons olive oil
½ cup grated cheddar cheese

● **Preheat the oven to 375°F. Generously butter a loaf pan, 8½ by 4½ by 2½ inches.**

Combine the soy flour, whey, eggs, baking powder, sour cream, and oil in a bowl and mix well. Fold in half of the cheddar. Pour the batter into the pan and sprinkle the remaining cheddar on top. Bake for 25 minutes, or until a tester comes out clean. Serve immediately or store, wrapped well in plastic wrap, in the refrigerator for up to 2 days or in the freezer for up to 1 month.

Makes 1 loaf

• Bacon Pepper Bread •

Serve this appetizing bread with eggs for breakfast or with a big salad for a light lunch.

> TOTAL CARBOHYDRATES:
>
> 18.8 grams per loaf

butter for greasing the loaf pan
1/3 cup soy flour (available at natural-food stores)
1/3 cup whey protein (available at natural-food stores)
2 large eggs
1/2 teaspoon baking powder
2 tablespoons sour cream
1/2 teaspoon freshly ground pepper
3 strips of bacon, cooked and crumbled

• **Preheat the oven to 375°F. Generously butter a loaf pan, 8½ by 4½ by 2½ inches.**

Combine the soy flour, whey, eggs, baking powder, sour cream, and pepper in a bowl and mix well. Fold in half of the bacon bits. Pour the batter into the prepared pan and sprinkle the remaining bacon on top. Bake for 25 minutes, or until a tester comes out clean. Serve immediately or store, wrapped well in plastic wrap, in the refrigerator for up to 2 days or in the freezer for up to 1 month.

Makes 1 loaf

• Sesame Sour Cream Muffins •

Go ahead—spread butter, cream cheese, or pâté on these savory muffins. You'll never miss the old white bread. They make a great accompaniment for soup or a salad.

> TOTAL CARBOHYDRATES: *15 grams*
>
> PER SERVING: *3.8 grams per muffin*

¼ cup tofu or soy flour
    (available at natural-
    food stores)
¼ cup ground sesame seeds
    (see Hint on page 190)

3 tablespoons sour cream
2 tablespoons butter, melted
½ teaspoon baking powder
2 large eggs, lightly beaten

● **Preheat oven to 350°F. Generously butter four ½-cup muffin tins.**

    Combine the flour, sesame seeds, sour cream, melted butter, baking powder, and eggs in a food processor and process for 2 to 3 minutes, or until smooth. Divide the batter evenly among the 4 muffin tins, filling each about half full. Fill the empty muffin tins with water. Bake for 20 to 25 minutes, or until a tester comes out clean. Let the muffins cool in the tins for 5 minutes, then turn them out onto a rack to cool completely.

Makes 4 muffins

• Savory Cheese Bites •

These appetizing crackers have a cookie-like texture. Serve them with soups and salads.

> TOTAL AVAILABLE CARBOHYDRATES: *25 grams*
>
> PER SERVING: *1.2 grams per "bite"*

butter for greasing the cookie sheet
¾ cup Atkins Bake Mix*
4 tablespoons (½ stick) butter
2 large egg whites
¼ cup sunflower seeds
⅓ cup grated Parmesan cheese
1 tablespoon lemon juice
1 tablespoon grated lemon zest
¼ teaspoon salt
½ teaspoon pepper
⅓ cup seltzer

• **Preheat the oven to 375°F. Generously butter a cookie sheet.**
  Combine the bake mix, butter, egg whites, sunflower seeds, Parmesan, lemon juice, lemon zest, salt, pepper, and seltzer in a large bowl and mix well, until smooth. Drop the batter by the heaping tablespoon on the prepared cookie sheet. Bake for 18 minutes, or until lightly golden. Remove from the oven and let cool slightly. Turn the cookies out onto a wire rack and let cool completely. Serve immediately or store in an airtight container for up to 5 days.

Makes about 20 "bites"

* Available through mail order by calling 1-888-DR ATKINS.

• Yorkshire Pudding •

A puffy, golden-brown Yorkshire pudding, baked here in individual ramekins, is a great accompaniment for Rib-eye Steak with Red Wine Sauce (page 129).

> TOTAL CARBOHYDRATES: *10.8 grams*
>
> PER SERVING: *5.4 grams*

butter for greasing the
    ramekins
1/4 cup soy flour

1/2 cup heavy cream
1/3 cup seltzer
2 large eggs

• **Preheat the oven to 450°F. Generously butter four 5-ounce ramekins.**

Beat together the flour, cream, seltzer, and eggs in a bowl with an electric mixer. Divide the batter among the prepared ramekins and bake for 18 to 20 minutes, or until puffed and golden.

Serves 4

• Butter Rum Muffins •

You'll hardly feel deprived when you sit down to a breakfast of these delicious muffins spread with butter and a hot cup of coffee (decaf, of course) with heavy cream.

> TOTAL CARBOHYDRATES: 19.8 grams
>
> PER SERVING: 5 grams per muffin

¼ cup tofu or soy flour (available at natural-food stores)

¼ cup ground sesame seeds (see Hint on page 190)

¼ cup whey protein (available at some natural-food stores)

2 large eggs, lightly beaten

3 tablespoons sour cream

1 tablespoon butter, softened

1 teaspoon rum

1½ packets sugar substitute (do not use Equal or aspartame; they lose their sweetness when heated)

½ teaspoon vanilla extract

½ teaspoon baking powder

• **Preheat oven to 350°F. Generously butter four ½-cup muffin tins.**

Combine the flour, sesame seeds, whey protein, eggs, sour cream, butter, rum, sugar substitute, vanilla extract, and baking powder in a food processor and process for 2 to 3 minutes, or until smooth. Divide the batter evenly among 4 muffin tins, filling each about half full, and fill empty muffin tins with water. Bake for 20 to 25 minutes, or until a tester comes out clean. Let the muffins cool in the tins for 5 minutes, then turn them out onto a rack to cool completely.

Variation: **For luscious homemade blueberry muffins, add ¼ cup of blueberries (5.1 grams carbohydrate)to the batter.**

Makes 4 muffins

• Breadings I, II, and III •

One afternoon Dr. Atkins and I decided to create the perfect low-carbohydrate coating. The results were so wonderful that we created three! They all work beautifully, so you can select the one you want to use, depending on the availability of ingredients.

Hint:

To grind pork rinds, place them in a food processor for 40 seconds.
To grind sesame seeds, place them in a food processor for 45 seconds.

Variations: For a different taste, add ½ teaspoon of dried herbs. Thyme, rosemary, and sage work well with meat, and tarragon is wonderful with chicken and fish. For a spicier coating, add cayenne pepper or dry mustard to taste.

• Breading I •

Pork Rind—Sesame Breading

> TOTAL CARBOHYDRATES:
> 7.1 grams per ¾ cup

½ cup ground pork rinds (see
    Hint on page 190)
½ teaspoon pepper

¼ cup ground sesame seeds
    (see Hint on page 190)

• Combine the pork rinds, pepper, and sesame seeds in a bowl and mix well. Use immediately or store in an airtight container for up to 1 week.

Makes about ¾ cup

• Breading II •

Sesame-Tofu Breading

> TOTAL CARBOHYDRATES:
> 14 grams per ½ cup

¼ cup ground sesame seeds
    (see Hint on page 190)
½ teaspoon pepper

¼ cup tofu or soy flour
    (available at natural-
    food stores)

• Combine the ground sesame seeds, pepper, and flour in a bowl and mix well. Use immediately or store in an airtight container for up to 1 week.

Makes about ½ cup

• Breading III •

Pork Rind—Tofu Breading

> TOTAL CARBOHYDRATES:
>
> *7.5 grams per ¾ cup*

½ cup ground pork rinds (see
    Hint on page 190)
¼ teaspoon pepper

¼ cup tofu or soy flour
    (available at natural-
    food stores)

•   **Combine the pork rinds, pepper, and flour in a bowl and mix
well. Use immediately or store in an airtight container for up to 1
week.**

Makes about ¾ cup

Desserts

•

Zabaglione

Swedish Cream

Coconut Custard Pudding

Chocolate Butter Cream

Hazelnut Torte

Crustless Cheesecake

Coconut Cookies

Shortcake Veronique with a Kiss of Rum

Dr. Atkins' Quick and Easy Dessert

· Zabaglione ·

This luxurious custard is fused with rich marsala wine and complemented by fresh berries. It is the perfect ending for a dinner or a brunch. Enjoy!

> TOTAL CARBOHYDRATES: *10.6 grams*
>
> PER SERVING: *5.3 grams*

4 egg yolks
1½ packets sugar substitute
    (do not use Equal or
    aspartame; they lose
    their sweetness when
    heated)

¼ cup dry marsala wine
¼ cup blueberries
2 large ripe strawberries
2 sprigs fresh mint leaves,
    washed and dried for
    garnish

• **Combine the egg yolks, sugar substitute, and marsala in a food processor and blend for about 15 seconds. Pour the mixture into the top of a double boiler over gently simmering water and whisk constantly for about 5 minutes, until it thickens to the consistency of whipped cream. Pour into 2 small bowls or ramekins. Garnish each with half of the blueberries, a strawberry, and a sprig of mint leaves. Serve or chill. The custard can be chilled and served for up to 3 days.**

Serves 2

• Swedish Cream •

Serve this sumptuous dessert on its own or with garnish of Ginger Syrup (page 207).

> **TOTAL CARBOHYDRATES:** *8.7 grams*
> **PER SERVING:** *4.35 grams*

½ cup heavy cream
⅓ envelope unflavored gelatin
1½ packets sugar substitute
    (do not use Equal or
    aspartame; they lose
    their sweetness when
    heated)

½ teaspoon vanilla extract
½ cup sour cream

• Combine ¼ cup of the cream and the gelatin in a small saucepan and cook over very low heat, whisking constantly, for 1 to 2 minutes, until the gelatin is dissolved. Slowly add the remaining cream, whisking constantly. Add the sugar substitute and vanilla extract, and cook for 10 minutes, whisking frequently. Cool to room temperature. Whisk in the sour cream until the cream is smooth. Serve at room temperature or chilled.

Makes about 1 cup

Variation: For a more piquant taste, add ½ teaspoon of grated lemon zest to the cream when adding the sour cream.

• Coconut Custard Pudding •

Rich and creamy, this coconut pudding has delicious butter-scotch undertones.

> TOTAL CARBOHYDRATES: *17.2 grams*
> PER SERVING: *8.6 grams*

one 14-ounce can unsweetened
    coconut milk
½ cup heavy cream
1 tablespoon butterscotch
    extract
3 egg yolks

2 packets different brands of
    sugar substitute or 3
    packets of the same kind
    (do not use Equal or
    aspartame; they lose
    their sweetness when
    heated) (see Note)

● Bring the coconut milk and heavy cream to a boil in a saucepan, then turn the heat to very low.

Meanwhile, whisk together the butterscotch extract, egg yolks, and sugar substitute in a bowl.

Whisk the egg mixture into the cream mixture, a little at a time, until incorporated. Simmer over very low heat, stirring constantly, for 5 minutes. Transfer the pan to a large bowl or sink filled with cold water and let cool for 5 minutes. Serve the pudding at room temperature or chilled.

Serves 2

Note: We suggest using a combination of substitute sugar sweeteners because when different types are used together, they have a synergistic effect. Therefore, less is needed.

• Chocolate Butter Cream •

This velvety chocolate cream tastes great either on its own, served in individual glass bowls, or as an accompaniment to Hazelnut Torte (page 199).

> TOTAL CARBOHYDRATES:
>
> 4.4 grams per cup

4 large egg yolks
2 tablespoons cognac
½ teaspoon vanilla extract
1 tablespoon shaved
    unsweetened dark
    chocolate
8 tablespoons (1 stick)
    unsalted butter, softened

1 packet sugar substitute (do
    not use Equal or
    aspartame; they lose
    their sweetness when
    heated)

• **Beat the egg yolks, cognac, vanilla extract, chocolate, butter, and sugar substitute in a large bowl with an electric mixer for 2 minutes. Place the mixture in the top of a double boiler over gently simmering water and cook it for 7 minutes, stirring constantly. Remove from the heat, let cool to room temperature, and serve.**

Makes about 1 cup or 2 servings

• *Hazelnut Torte* •

This baked hazelnut torte has a rich flavor and a wonderful aroma. Serve with whipped cream or Chocolate Butter Cream (page 198).

> TOTAL CARBOHYDRATES: *21.8 grams*
>
> PER SERVING: *5.5–7.4 grams*

butter for greasing the pan

¾ cup plus 2 tablespoons ground hazelnuts

1 tablespoon whey protein (available at natural-food stores)

2 large eggs

1 tablespoon sour cream

1 packet sugar substitute (do not use Equal or aspartame; they lose their sweetness when heated)

½ tablespoon baking powder

- **Preheat the oven to 350°F.**

    Generously butter an 8-inch round cake pan and sprinkle the 2 tablespoons of hazelnuts over the bottom of the pan.

    Combine the remaining hazelnuts, whey protein, eggs, sour cream, sugar substitute, and baking powder in a large bowl. Using an electric mixer, blend at medium-high speed about 2 minutes, until fluffy. Pour the batter into the prepared pan. Bake for 25 minutes, or until a tester comes out clean. Cool to room temperature and serve.

Serves 3 or 4

• Crustless Cheesecake •

There's no need to give up rich, luscious desserts while you're on the Atkins diet. Here's a sublime crustless cheesecake that is sure to delight sweet teeth everywhere.

> TOTAL CARBOHYDRATES: *21 grams*
>
> PER SERVING: *2.6 grams*

12 ounces cream cheese, softened
2 packets different sugar substitutes or 3 packets of the same kind (see Note)
1 teaspoon vanilla extract
1 cup heavy cream
½ cup fresh strawberries, quartered (optional / 5.2 grams of carbohydrate)

• Combine the cream cheese, sugar substitute, and vanilla extract in a bowl and mix well. Beat the heavy cream in a bowl until it forms soft peaks. Fold the whipped cream into the cream cheese mixture.

Transfer the mixture to a large glass bowl and chill, covered with plastic wrap, for at least 25 minutes. Top with the berries, if using. Serve immediately or store, covered with plastic wrap, in the refrigerator for up to 2 days.

Serves 8

Note: We suggest using a combination of artificial sweeteners because when different types are used together, they have a synergistic effect. Therefore, less is needed.

• Coconut Cookies •

Yes, you can indulge in fresh-baked cookies! These nutty clusters are a marvelous treat. When baking the cookies, be sure to leave plenty of room around them so they can spread out.

> TOTAL AVAILABLE CARBOHYDRATES: *19.3 grams*
>
> PER SERVING: *.9 per cookie*

butter for greasing the cookie
  sheet
½ cup Atkins Bake Mix*
¼ cup shredded unsweetened
  coconut
¼ cup coarsely chopped
  hazelnuts
2 egg whites
2 tablespoons seltzer

8 tablespoons butter (1 stick),
  softened
2 packets different sugar
  substitute or 3 packets of
  the same kind (do not
  use Equal or aspartame;
  they lose their sweetness
  when heated) (see Note)

* Preheat oven to 375°F.
  Generously butter a cookie sheet.
  Combine the bake mix, coconut, hazelnuts, egg whites, seltzer, butter, and sugar substitute in a bowl and mix well. Drop the batter by rounded tablespoons onto the prepared cookie sheet (you will have about 20). Bake for 20 minutes, or until lightly golden. Remove from the oven and cool slightly. Serve immediately or store in an airtight container for up to 1 week.

Makes about 20 cookies

Note: We suggest using a combination of sugar substitutes because when different types are used together, they have a synergistic effect. Therefore, less is needed.

* Available through mail order by calling 1-888-DR ATKINS.

• Shortcake Veronique •
with a Kiss of Rum

No one will believe that this dessert is part of a diet. The rum adds a depth of flavor that is perfectly complemented by the fresh berries.

> TOTAL CARBOHYDRATES: *16.9 grams*
>
> PER SERVING: *8.5 grams*

2 butter rum muffins (recipe on page 189), halved
2 teaspoons rum (do not substitute liqueurs, because they are high in sugar)

½ cup heavy cream
1 packet sugar substitute
2 large strawberries, halved

• Sprinkle the muffin halves with the rum. Combine the cream and sugar substitute in a bowl and beat until soft peaks form. Divide the whipped cream among the muffin halves. Place a strawberry half in the center of each shortcake half. Serve immediately.

Serves 2

· Dr. Atkins' Quick · and Easy Dessert

When I don't have time to make a dessert, I will invariably find Dr. Atkins in the kitchen improvising a sweet finale. This is one of his best concoctions.

> TOTAL CARBOHYDRATES: *11.9 grams*
>
> PER SERVING: *6 grams*

2 coconut cookies (recipe on page 201) or ¼ cup shredded unsweetened coconut
¼ cup sour cream
¼ cup heavy cream

2 large strawberries, sliced
2 packets different sugar substitutes or 3 packets of the same kind (see Note)*
a dash of rum or cognac

- **Divide the cookies, crumbled, or the coconut between 2 small serving bowls. Top each serving with half of the sour cream, half of the heavy cream, half of the strawberries, half of the sugar substitute, and a sprinkling of rum. Serve immediately.**

Serves 2

Note: **We suggest using a combination of artificial sweeteners because when different types are used together, they have a synergistic effect. Therefore, less is needed.**

* Although most published scientific studies have proclaimed aspartame (NutraSweet, Equal) to be safe, clinical experience has often indicated otherwise. Headaches, irritability, and failure to lose weight or to control blood glucose have all been reported, as well as cross reactions in those who cannot tolerate monosodium glutamate (MSG). Consult with your local doctor if you have any concern about your use of aspartame. The best advice may be to use it sparingly, preferably blending it with other sweeteners. Remember, too, that aspartame loses its sweetness when heated.

Beverages

•

Ginger Syrup
Homemade Ginger Ale
Ginger Cream
Warm Spiced Cocktail

• Ginger Syrup •

This fragrant ginger syrup can be used to make homemade ginger ale. It is also delicious when drizzled on Coconut Custard Pudding (page 197) or whipped with heavy cream.

> TOTAL CARBOHYDRATES:
>
> 6 grams per 1½ cups

one 3-inch piece of fresh
    gingerroot, peeled and
    cut into 1-inch pieces
2 cups water
juice of ½ lemon
2 teaspoons vanilla extract

3 packets different sugar
    substitutes or 4 packets
    of the same kind (do not
    use Equal or aspartame;
    they lose their sweetness
    when heated) (see Note)

● **Combine the gingerroot, water, lemon juice, vanilla extract, and sugar substitute in a saucepan. Bring to a gentle boil and simmer, covered, for 20 minutes. Strain into a bowl through a sieve lined with a double thickness of rinsed and squeezed cheesecloth, pressing down on the solids with the back of a spoon. Add additional sugar substitute or vanilla extract, to taste.**

Makes about 1½ cups

Note: We suggest using a combination of artificial sweeteners because when different types are used together, they have a synergistic effect. Therefore, less is needed.

• Homemade Ginger Ale •

This tasty ginger ale can be made to varying degrees of strength.
Simply adjust the amounts of ginger syrup and seltzer.

TOTAL CARBOHYDRATES:

1.3 grams per ¾ cup

⅓ cup ginger syrup (page
  207)
½ cup cold seltzer

ice
mint leaves for garnish
  (optional)

- **Combine the ginger syrup, seltzer, and ice in a tall glass. Stir gently and garnish with the mint leaves if desired. Serve immediately.**

Makes about ¾ cup

• Ginger Cream •

Serve this rich, creamy dessert drink in chilled martini glasses.

> TOTAL CARBOHYDRATES: *11.6 grams*
>
> PER SERVING: *5.8 grams*

½ cup ginger syrup (page 207)

1½ cups very cold heavy cream

2 strips orange zest for garnish (optional)

dash of cinnamon, or to taste, for garnish (optional)

• **Thoroughly blend together the ginger syrup and cream in a bowl or small pitcher. Pour into 2 chilled glasses and garnish each with a strip of orange zest and a dusting of cinnamon if desired. Serve immediately.**

Makes about 2 cups

• Warm Spiced Cocktail

This tasty beverage makes a comforting, nonalcoholic aperitif, especially on a chilly evening.

> TOTAL CARBOHYDRATES: *2.8 grams*
>
> PER SERVING: *1.4 grams*

2 cups beef broth
4 teaspoons tomato sauce
½ teaspoon grated onion
1 teaspoon Worcestershire sauce

½ teaspoon drained horseradish
1 or 2 drops hot pepper sauce, or to taste
salt and pepper to taste

• **Stir together the broth, tomato sauce, onion, Worcestershire sauce, horseradish, hot pepper sauce, salt, and pepper in a small saucepan. Heat over medium heat, stirring occasionally, until warmed through. Divide between 2 mugs and serve.**

Serves 2

Quick and Easy Low-Carbohydrate Food List

PROTEINS

BEEF

ALL CHEESES*

(AGED)

Blue cheeses
Brie
Camembert
Cheddar
Feta
Fontina
Goat cheeses
Gouda
Gruyère
Havarti
Monterey Jack
Mozzarella
Muenster
Parmigiano
Provolone
Romano
Sardo
Swiss

(FRESH)

Cottage
Cream
Farmer
Goat
Mascarpone
Pot
Ricotta

* For cheeses you should avoid,
see Hidden Carbohydrates on
pages 20–21.

CHICKEN
DUCK
EGGS
ALL FISH
(INCLUDING CANNED)

Anchovy
Bass
Bluefish
Catfish
Cod
Flounder
Monk
Red snapper
Salmon
Sardines
Scrod
Sole
Swordfish
Trout
Tuna
Whitefish

SHELLFISH

Clams
Crab
Crawfish
Lobster
Mussels
Oysters
Scallops
Shrimp
Squid

GAME BIRDS
LAMB
MILK PRODUCTS
Butter
Cream
Sour cream
Whipped cream

PORK
RABBIT
TURKEY
VEAL
VENISON

SALAD
VEGETABLES
AND GREENS

Alfalfa sprouts
Arugula
Bean sprouts
Bokchoy
Cabbage
Celery
Chicory
Chinese cabbage
Chives
Collard greens
Cucumber
Endive
Escarole
Fennel
Jicama
Kale
Leeks
Lettuce
Mushrooms
Mustard greens

Okra
Peppers
Radishes
Sorrel
Spinach
Swiss chard
Watercress

OTHER
LOW-CARBOHYDRATE
VEGETABLES

Artichoke
Asparagus
Avocado
Broccoli
Broccoli rabe
Brussels sprouts
Cauliflower
Eggplant
Kohlrabi
Onions
Plantains
Pumpkin
Rhubarb
Sauerkraut
Scallions
Snow peas
Spaghetti squash
String/green beans
Turnips
Water chestnuts
Zucchini

HERBS
Basil
Bay leaf
Chervil

Chives
Cilantro
Dill
Lemon grass
Marjoram
Mint
Oregano
Parsley
Rosemary
Sage
Tarragon
Thyme

NUTS AND SEEDS

Almonds
Brazil nuts
Coconut (fresh)
Filberts (hazelnuts)
Macadamias
Pecans
Pine nuts (pignoli)
Pumpkin seeds
Sesame seeds
Sunflower seeds
Walnuts

FATS AND OILS
(Cold-pressed oils are preferred.)

Animal fat
Butter
Canola oil
Mayonnaise
Olive oil
Safflower oil
Sesame oil
Soybean oil
Sunflower oil
Walnut oil

FLOUR AND "BREADINGS"

Atkins Bake Mix
Pork rinds
Soy flour
Tofu flour
Whey protein

SUGAR SUBSTITUTES

Each dieter must determine the sweeteners that agree with him or her.* The most efficient way to use sweeteners is to use more than one type together because sweeteners create a synergistic effect. You should experiment with combinations until you discover your favorite and the amount to use for desired sweetness.

*Although most published scientific studies have proclaimed aspartame (NutraSweet, Equal) to be safe, clinical experience has often indicated otherwise. Headaches, irritability, and failure to lose weight or to control blood glucose have all been reported, as well as cross reactions in those who cannot tolerate monosodium glutamate (MSG). Consult with your local doctor if you have any concern about your use of aspartame. The best advice may be to use it sparingly, preferably blending it with other sweeteners. Remember, too, that aspartame loses its sweetness when heated.

• Acknowledgments •

A VERY SPECIAL THANKS TO . . .

My sister, Valentina Zimbalkin, whose culinary talents I have always admired and secretly envied.

Our friend Anya Senoret, whose creativity extends from designing beautiful clothes to creating wonderful dishes.

Nena, who was visiting from Croatia.

My niece and nephew, Tina and Michael (eight and ten years old), who were my "official tasters" and whose verdicts of "cool" and "awesome" were very encouraging.

My former roommate, Stella Siu, who gave me some wonderful pointers.

Kathleen Duffy Freud, Bettina Newman, and Michael Cohn for their expertise and assistance.

My editors at Simon & Schuster, Fred Hills and Sydny Miner, for their faith and support under daunting deadlines.

Erika Sommer, my coauthor, without whom this book would not have been born.

Nancy Hancock, last but not least, who convinced Simon & Schuster that this book "needed to be!"

Want the latest breakthroughs and news?
Come visit us on the web at: www.atkinscenter.com.

Call toll-free 1-888-DR-ATKINS (1-888-372-8546)
to order Atkins products or to find a retailer near you
that carries them.

If you enjoyed *Dr. Atkins' Quick & Easy New Diet
Cookbook* and would like to learn more,
you might also want to read:

Dr. Atkins' Age-Defying Diet Revolution

Eat well and stay young! Dr. Atkins, using thirty years of experience with nutrition and the latest scientific breakthroughs, has created a new Age-Defying Diet. Using this simple program you can . . . defy your age!

Dr. Atkins' New Diet Revolution, Revised and Updated

The #1 best-selling book that started it all! Includes new chapters and information about this revolutionary weight loss program.

Dr. Atkins' Vita-Nutrient Solution

A comprehensive guide to more than 120 supplements, including vitamins, minerals, amino acids, and herbs.

How to Learn More About the Atkins Center

Established in 1970, the Atkins Center for Complementary Medicine is an eighty-staff, six-story medical facility in the heart of New York City. The Atkins Center's mission is to first address major health disorders through vita-nutrient therapies, diet modifications, and lifestyle changes that can enhance the body's own restorative powers before patients resort to prescription drugs and/or surgical procedures. More than sixty thousand patients have been treated at the Atkins Center for a wide variety of disorders, including cancer, arthritis, asthma, diabetes, heart/cardiovascular disease, chronic fatigue, multiple sclerosis, as well as weight problems.

For information on becoming a patient at the Atkins Center,
please call 1-888-ATKINS-8 (1-888-285-4678).

ABOUT THE AUTHORS

ROBERT C. ATKINS, M.D., is the founder and medical director of the Atkins Center for Complementary Medicine. A 1951 graduate of the University of Michigan, he received his medical degree from Cornell University Medical School in 1955, and went on to specialize in cardiology. He has been a practicing physician for over thirty years and is the author of several books. As a leader in the areas of natural medicine and nutritional pharmacology, he has built an international reputation. He is the recipient of the World Organization of Alternative Medicine's Recognition of Achievement Award and was the National Health Federation's Man of the Year. His many media appearances, where he has discussed diet and health, include "Larry King Live," "Oprah," "CBS This Morning," and "CNBC," among others. Many magazine and newspaper articles have featured his work, and he also has a nationally syndicated radio show. Dr. Atkins is the editor of his own national monthly newsletter, "Dr. Atkins' Health Revelations." He lives in New York City with his wife, Veronica.

VERONICA ATKINS was born in Russia and narrowly escaped the Nazi onslaught during World War II by fleeing to live with her great-aunt in Vienna. In the years since, she has lived in seven countries and become fluent in as many languages. Her far-flung travels have given her an extensive knowledge of international cuisine. Music has also played an important role in her life. She began singing in Europe at a young age and performed professionally as an opera singer from 1963 to 1976. Today she is actively involved in Dr. Atkins' work at the Center for Complementary Medicine. She serves on the board of directors of the Foundation for the Advancement of Innovative Medicine Education group. Her current stage is the kitchen, where she actively creates and develops delicious low-carbohydrate recipes.